Management of common health problems of drug users

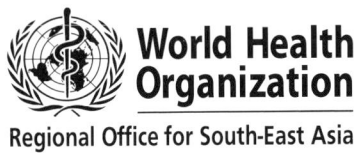

Regional Office for South-East Asia

WHO Library Cataloguing-in-Publication data

World Health Organization, Regional Office for South-East Asia.

Management of common health problems of drug users.

(Technical Publication Series No. 56)

1. Substance Abuse, Intravenous drug therapy prevention and control. 2. Drug Utilization.
3. Substance-Related Disorders. 4. Primary Health Care education.
5. Communicable Diseases complications - therapy. 6. Manuals.

ISBN   978-92-9022-292-7   (NLM classification: WB330)

This publication is available on the Internet at www.searo.who.int/hiv-aids publications.

Copies may be requested from the HIV Unit, Department of Communicable Diseases, World Health Organization, Regional Office for South-East Asia, Indraprastha Estate, Mahatma Gandhi Marg, New Delhi 110 002, India, e-mail: hiv@searo.who.int.

© World Health Organization 2009

All rights reserved. Requests for publications, or for permission to reproduce or translate WHO publications – whether for sale or for noncommercial distribution – can be obtained from Publishing and Sales, World Health Organization, Regional Office for South-East Asia, Indraprastha Estate, Mahatma Gandhi Marg, New Delhi 110 002, India (fax: +91 11 23370197; e-mail: publications@searo.who.int. The designations employed and the presentation of the material in this publication do not imply the expression of any opinion whatsoever on the part of the World Health Organization concerning the legal status of any country, territory, city or area or of its authorities, or concerning the delimitation of its frontiers or boundaries. Dotted lines on maps represent approximate border lines for which there may not yet be full agreement. The mention of specific companies or of certain manufacturers' products does not imply that they are endorsed or recommended by the World Health Organization in preference to others of a similar nature that are not mentioned. Errors and omissions excepted, the names of proprietary products are distinguished by initial capital letters. All reasonable precautions have been taken by the World Health Organization to verify the information contained in this publication. However, the published material is being distributed without warranty of any kind, either expressed or implied. The responsibility for the interpretation and use of the material lies with the reader. In no event shall the World Health Organization be liable for damages arising from its use.

This publication contains the collective views of an international group of experts and does not necessarily represent the decisions or the stated policy of the World Health Organization.

Printed in India

Contents

Acknowledgements		iv
Preface		v
Acronyms and abbreviations		vii
1.	INTRODUCTION	1
1.1	What are drugs?	1
1.2	Drug use in Asia	2
1.3	Drugs that are commonly injected in Asia	3
1.4	Profile of drug users in Asia	5
1.5	Primary health-care services for drug users	6
1.6	Models for delivery of primary health care to drug users	7
1.7	Comprehensive service package for drug users	9
2.	COMMON HEALTH PROBLEMS ASSOCIATED WITH DRUG USE/INJECTING DRUG USE	11
2.1	Injection-related injuries	12
2.2	Injection-related infections	14
2.3	Complications of injection-related infections	19
2.4	Infectious diseases	28
2.5	Non-infectious disorders	79
2.6	Other common medical problems	102
3.	UNIVERSAL PRECAUTIONS IN THE PRIMARY HEALTH-CARE SETTING	108
3.1	Universal precautions	108
3.2.	Post-exposure prophylaxis (PEP)	108

Annex 1: Principles for establishing services for drug users	113
Annex 2: Operational issues: staff, facilities and equipment	116
Annex 3: Antibiotics used to treat infections in drug users	121
Annex 4: Sample educational materials for injecting drug users	123
References	126

Acknowledgements

The World Health Organization (WHO) Regional Office for South-East Asia expresses its gratitude to M. Suresh Kumar (Chennai, India) and Nick Walsh (Public Health Consultant, Melbourne, Australia) for preparing these guidelines for the World Health Organization.

These guidelines used the following publications as key references: *Guidelines for primary health care services for injecting drug users*, developed by the Ministry of Health, Myanmar and WHO Yangon, and published in October 2005; and *Management of HIV infection and antiretroviral therapy in adults and adolescents: a clinical manual*, New Delhi, WHO Regional Office for South-East Asia, 2007.

These guidelines were developed based on discussions held with health-care workers, researchers and programme managers from South-East Asia during a regional consultation organized by the World Health Organization Regional Office for South-East Asia in New Delhi during 2006. This consultation meeting reviewed the data on and experiences of implementing harm-reduction services for drug users in the Region.

We thank the following for their comments and contributions: Lokendra Rai, Nepal; Robert Kosasih, Indonesia; Ashita Mittal, United Nations Office for Drug and Crime, Regional Office for South-Asia (UNODC), New Delhi, India; Keisam Priyokumar, Jawahar Lal Nehru Hospital, Imphal, India; Hans-Guenter Meyer-Thompson, GTZ; Philippe Clevenbergh, The Union's Office in Myanmar; Oscar Barreneche, WHO Country Office Myanmar; Po-Lin Chan and Suvanand Sahu, WHO Country Office, New Delhi, India; David Jacka and Sabine Flessenkaemper, WHO Country Office, Jakarta, Indonesia; Ying-Ru Lo and Annette Verster, WHO Headquarters, Geneva.

This work was coordinated by Mukta Sharma (WHO Regional Office for South-East Asia). The document was edited by Bandana Malhotra, and designed and typeset by Netra Shyam.

Preface

The World Health Organization (WHO) defines health as a "state of complete physical, mental and social well-being and not merely the absence of disease or infirmity" and this is a fundamental human right. This right to health applies as much to drug users as to any other population. Yet, provision of primary health-care services to this group remains inadequate and is further compounded by marginalization, stigmatization and harassment from the wider community. The threat of imprisonment or other penalties and poverty also contribute to poor access to mainstream health services. Many drug users do not have reliable access to accurate health information and have specific needs that are sometimes beyond the capacity of regular health services.

Primary health-care services aim to provide a practical approach to making essential health care universally accessible to individuals and families in the community in an acceptable and affordable way, and with their full participation. These services should be delivered by health-care providers who understand the health priorities of the communities they serve, and have the confidence and trust of their clients. As such, primary health care should include a broad range of services required to meet the multiple health needs of people who use drugs. Greater access to primary health-care services sensitive to the needs of drug users can reduce inpatient hospitalization, health costs and the burden on existing mainstream health services. It is thus important to provide early interventions that utilize different health-care approaches to target and reach this largely hidden population.

Primary health care for drug users aims to promote health by providing a comprehensive harm-reduction package including outreach; peer-led interventions; information, education and communication; condoms; sterile injection equipment; and effective drug treatment including opioid substitution therapy. It also aims to reduce morbidity and mortality among all drug users by early identification and treatment of infections and other drug use-related illnesses; and provide care, treatment and support for HIV-infected drug users.

These clinical guidelines are intended for use by doctors, nurses and other health-care workers who work in community outreach, drop-in centres, community clinics, drug treatment centres, prison clinics, and primary- and secondary-level hospitals. They offer guidance on the provision of primary health care to drug users and focus on the clinical management of common medical problems associated with drug use, in particular, injecting drug use in the presence or absence of HIV infection. These guidelines should be considered along with others developed by the WHO, United Nations Office on Drugs and Crime (UNODC) and Family Health International/United States Agency for International Development (FHI/USAID) on providing treatment and care for substance-using populations.

Acronyms and abbreviations

AFB	acid-fast bacilli
AIDS	acquired immune deficiency syndrome
ALT	alanine aminotransferase
ART	antiretroviral therapy
ARV	antiretroviral (drug)
ASO	AIDS Service Organization
ATS	amphetamine-type stimulants
BBV	bloodborne virus
CBO	community-based organization
CBT	cognitive–behavioural therapy
CITC	client-initiated testing and counselling
CMV	cytomegalovirus
CPR	cardiopulmonary resuscitation
CXR	chest X-ray
DIC	drop-in centre
DNA	deoxyribonucleic acid
DOTS	directly observed treatment, short-course
DU	drug user
ELISA	enzyme-linked immunosorbent assay
EPTB	extrapulmonary tuberculosis
GC/CT	gonococcal infection/*Chlamydia trachomatis*
GUD	genital ulcer disease
HBeAg	hepatitis B e antigen
HbsAb	antibody to hepatitis B surface antigen
HBsAg	hepatitis B surface antigen
HBV	hepatitis B virus
HCV	hepatitis C virus
HIV	human immunodeficiency virus
HSV-2	herpes simplex virus-2
ICU	intensive care unit
IDU	injecting drug user
IEC	information, education and communication

IFN	interferon
IM	intramuscular
INH	isoniazid
IPT	isoniazid preventive therapy
IRIS	immune reconstitution inflammatory syndrome
IV	intravenous
LGV	lymphogranuloma venereum
MAC	*Mycobacterium avium* complex
MDMA	methylenedioxymethamphetamine
MDR	multidrug-resistant
MRSA	methicillin-resistant *Staphylococcus aureus*
MTCT	mother-to-child transmission
NGO	nongovernmental organization
NSAID	non-steroidal anti-inflammatory drug
OI	opportunistic infection
ORS	oral rehydration solution
OST	opioid substitution therapy
OTC	over the counter
PCP	*Pneumocystis jiroveci* pneumonia (earlier known as *Pneumocystis carinii*)
PEG-IFN	pegylated interferon
PEP	post-exposure prophylaxis
PGL	persistent generalized lymphadenopathy
PHCS	primary health-care service
PI	protease inhibitor
PID	pelvic inflammatory disease
PITC	provider-initiated testing and counselling
PLHIV	people living with HIV
PMTCT	prevention of mother-to-child transmission (of HIV)
PPD	purified protein derivative
PTB	pulmonary tuberculosis
SP	Spasmoproxyvon®
SSRI	selective serotonin reuptake inhibitor
STI	sexually transmitted infection
TB	tuberculosis
TLC	total lymphocyte count
TMP–SMX	trimethoprim–sulfamethoxazole
TT	tetanus toxoid
UNODC	United Nations Office on Drugs and Crime
WHO	World Health Organization

Introduction

1.1 What are drugs?

It is important to know what we understand and mean by the word drugs. People often have a different understanding of what drugs are and how they are classified. The *Lexicon of alcohol and drug terms* published by the WHO defines these terms as given below:[1]

DRUG

This is a term with varied usage. In medicine, it refers to any substance with the potential to prevent or cure disease or enhance physical or mental welfare and, in pharmacology, to any chemical agent that alters the biochemical and physiological processes of tissues or organisms. Hence, a drug is a substance that is, or could be, listed in a pharmacopoeia.

In common usage, the term often refers specifically to psychoactive drugs, and often, even more specifically, to illicit drugs, of which there is non-medical use in addition to any medical use.

PSYCHOACTIVE DRUG OR SUBSTANCE

This is a substance that, when ingested, affects mental processes, e.g. cognition or affect. This term and its equivalent, psychotropic drug, are the most neutral and descriptive terms for the whole class of substances, licit and illicit, of interest to drug policy. "Psychoactive" does not necessarily imply dependence-producing and, in common parlance, the term is often left unstated, as in "drug use" or "substance use".

Common usage distinguishes between licit and illicit drugs:
(1) Legal (licit) drugs include medicines, tobacco, alcohol and coffee/tea.

(2) Illegal (illicit) drugs are substances such as opium, heroin, cocaine, amphetamine-type stimulants (ATS), and cannabis (note: cannabis is an illicit drug in most countries in Asia but is a licit drug in countries such as Italy, Luxembourg, Portugal and Spain where personal cannabis use has been decriminalized).

1.2 Drug use in Asia

The use of opium, cannabis and hashish has historically been common throughout Asia. The use of heroin has been widespread since the 1980s. The past two decades have also seen widespread diffusion of injecting drug use, involving not only heroin but other synthetic opioids and other substances. Buprenorphine, a type of opioid that has sedative and pain-relieving effects, is reportedly used in India, Pakistan, Bangladesh, Nepal, Iran and China (less in China). Dextropropoxyphene (a common brand known as Spasmoproxyvon®* [SP]) is widely used in the North-Eastern Indian states. Most countries in Asia also report using mixed pharmaceuticals such as analgesics, antihistamines and tranquillizers. Solvents and glues are used by adolescents and children in India, Lao PDR, Indonesia, Mongolia, Viet Nam, the Philippines and Thailand.[2]

Since the late 1990s, ATS has increasingly become a drug of choice in Thailand, South Korea, Philippines, Taiwan, China, Japan, Cambodia, Lao PDR and Indonesia. The use of Ecstasy (methylenedioxymethamphetamine [MDMA]), a type of ATS, has become common in the dance party scene in Asia.

Polysubstance use and "cocktailing" of drugs is widespread in the Region. Pooling of money to purchase drugs and sharing of needles is common in Asia. There has been a marked increase in polydrug use for several reasons, such as when certain commonly used drugs are more difficult to access, often because drug seizures result in price increases. In such situations, it is common for substance users to seek and use a range of alternatives to achieve the desired effect.

---

*Manufactured by Wockhardt Ltd., India (dicyclomine 10 mg, dextropropoxyphene 65 mg, paracetamol 400 mg)

Introduction

MODES OF DRUG CONSUMPTION

Drugs can be taken by smoking, snorting, ingesting (eating, drinking) or injecting. Not all drugs can be taken by all routes. It is important to note that people can switch from one method of taking drugs to another (e.g. from smoking to injecting heroin). Some people also take a number of different drugs by different routes over a period of time (e.g. drinking alcohol, smoking tobacco, swallowing Ecstasy or injecting heroin).

- *Drugs that are commonly smoked or inhaled* include tobacco, marijuana, opium, heroin, ATS and glue.
- *Drugs that are "chased" include heroin* – it is placed on foil and heated and turns into a sticky liquid which wriggles around like a Chinese dragon. Fumes are given off and inhaled through a tube, rolled up newspaper or magazine.
- *Drugs that are commonly ingested or swallowed* (as in drinking) include alcohol, opium, marijuana, sedatives (e.g. diazepam), ATS and heroin (rarely).
- Cocaine is commonly snorted (inhaling into the nostril).
- *Drugs that are commonly injected* include heroin, sedatives, ATS (less commonly) and buprenorphine.

1.3 Drugs that are commonly injected in Asia

HEROIN

Where heroin is the drug of choice in various countries of the Mekong Region, the favoured method of administration is injecting. The rate of heroin injecting does, however, vary from place to place, and in different cultural and social settings: once the initial phase of smoking and inhalation of heroin has generally passed, the data suggest that around 50–60% of heroin users inject.[2-5]

BUPRENORPHINE

Injecting buprenorphine is common in South Asia. Buprenorphine produced in India is diverted to the illicit drug market. A study of drug-sharing and injecting networks in Bangladesh found most IDUs in Bangladesh inject buprenorphine, with sharing of equipment and drugs. Poorer users tended to report larger, more open drug-sharing networks.[6]

AMPHETAMINE-TYPE STIMULANTS (ATS)

ATS are generally ingested or smoked, but injecting of ATS, albeit in smaller numbers, has been identified in Thailand, China, Lao PDR and Cambodia.[7,8] As a street drug, amphetamines are usually sold as a powder which contains amphetamine that has been mixed with other powders or drugs.

PROXYVON®

Proxyvon®* and Spasmoproxyvon® contain dextropoxyphene, a synthetic opiate which is produced legally and sold over the counter (OTC). Its street name is "Spasmo" or "SP". It costs approximately one tenth of the price of heroin and is therefore used as a substitute. Spasmoproxyvon® is commonly injected by IDUs in North-East India (Mizoram, Manipur and Nagaland).

MIDAZOLAM TABLETS

Midazolam, a short-acting benzodiazepine, is increasingly being used as a drug of injection in Bangkok. Midazolam tablets are crushed, dissolved in water, filtered and injected. Sharing of equipment is common. Abscesses, gangrene and vein degradation are common complications of such injecting.[9]

Most people do not start off their drug-using careers via injecting. However, due the efficiency of injecting in delivering a substance directly into the bloodstream and the lack of drug wastage, many DUs facing increased tolerance and financial pressures switch to this mode over time. A frequent practice in many countries is the sharing of one needle between many injectors. HIV and hepatitis C spread most rapidly among IDUs when such sharing of injecting paraphernalia occurs. Notably, it is not drug use that causes HIV infection, or even drug injecting; but the sharing of contaminated injecting equipment that transmits HIV infection.

Professional injectors (those who receive payment for injecting a client with an illicit drug) operate in Myanmar, Pakistan, India, Bangladesh, Nepal,

---

*Manufactured by Wockhardt Ltd., India (dextropropoxyphene 65 mg, paracetamol 400 mg)

Introduction

Viet Nam and Malaysia. Professional injectors rarely employ hygienic practices and consequently HIV transmission among IDUs is inevitable.

1.4 Profile of drug users in Asia

Drug use in Asia remains a phenomenon which is entrenched in poverty and marginalization. Most drug users are male. There appears to be an increasing trend towards a decreasing age at initiation of drug use. Cambodia, Lao PDR and Viet Nam report substantial populations of street children, who increasingly consume drugs, and live precariously with little or no family support or guardians. A substantial proportion of illicit DUs are unemployed or underemployed, and, while educational standards vary, large proportions have achieved lower secondary education at best.

DRUG USE AMONG WOMEN

Drug use among women in Asia is often considered a minor problem, with the number of women classified as IDUs estimated at 10% or less.[2] It has been suggested, however, that this figure may increase and that improved monitoring of the situation is required. In China, most IDUs are men but the number of women using drugs is increasing. In Yunnan and Guangxi provinces, women make up 16–25% of all IDUs in treatment and tend to be younger than male IDUs. Other countries in Asia where there are significant numbers of women IDUs include Nepal, India, Pakistan, Bangladesh, Indonesia, Viet Nam, Thailand, Sri Lanka, the Philippines, Taiwan, Japan and Malaysia.

In general:
- Women DUs are more likely to have a male sexual partner who injects drugs.
- Women tend to be introduced to drugs by husbands/boyfriends or other male members of their family.
- Access to drugs usually occurs through a male sexual partner.
- Women are more likely to share needles and to be injected by someone else.
- Women experience difficulty in avoiding drug use, and abstaining from and accessing drug treatment if the male partner is an active drug user.

FEMALE SEX WORKERS AND INJECTING DRUG USE

In Asia, studies have shown an overlap between sex work and injecting drug use, with approximately half of female IDUs estimated to sell sex.[10,11] This has been noted particularly in Viet Nam, parts of North-East India and China. In Guangxi province in China, 80% of female DUs sell sex. Female IDUs may become involved in sex work to pay for drugs. At the same time, sex workers may also use drugs. In some situations, brothel owners introduce sex workers to drugs. Women who are coerced or sold into sex work may also resort to drug use.

1.5 Primary health-care services for drug users

WHO defines health as a "state of complete physical, mental and social well-being and not merely the absence of disease or infirmity" and this is a fundamental human right.[12] As such, primary health care should include a broad range of services required to meet the multiple health needs of DUs.

The objectives of primary health care for DUs include the following:
- Promote health among DUs by providing a comprehensive harm-reduction package including: outreach; peer-led interventions; information, education and communication (IEC); condoms; sterile injection equipment; effective drug treatment, e.g. opioid substitution therapy (OST).
- Reduce morbidity and mortality among all DUs by early identification and treatment of infections and other drug use-related illnesses; and
- Provide HIV care, treatment and support for HIV-infected DUs.

Primary health-care services (PHCS) aim to provide a practical approach to making essential health care universally accessible to individuals and families in the community in an acceptable and affordable way, and with their full participation. These services should be delivered by health-care providers who understand the health priorities of the communities they serve, and have the confidence and trust of their clients.

Some of the barriers to DUs accessing services include the following:
- Drug use is illegal, so DUs often stay hidden and are reluctant to access health-care services.

Introduction

- Services are located far away from where DUs live or congregate to use substances.
- Stigma and discrimination towards DUs is prevalent in the community and among health-care workers due to:
  - Lack of knowledge among health-care providers on how to deal with DUs
  - Cultural differences between patients and service providers
  - Poor patient–physician communication
  - Lack of mutual trust, respect and confidentiality
  - Lack of knowledge in the community that drug dependence is a health problem rather than a moral or social problem.
- There is a lack of comprehensive services catering to the multiple needs of DUs. Families and communities do not know how to appropriately and effectively support DUs.
- Most DUs live in poverty, which further restricts their access to health care.

Barriers to access can be addressed by the following:
- Services should be close to the community or brought to the community through reaching out to the most vulnerable among DUs (e.g. women, adolescents, unemployed persons, slum dwellers, refugees and ethnic minorities).
- Involving former DUs or active DUs as staff members or patient advocates makes services more user-friendly.
- A range of essential services should be delivered appropriately to DUs. Families and communities should be trained and involved in caring and supporting substance-using individuals.
- Services should be offered free of cost or at subsidized rates.

1.6 Models for delivery of primary health care to drug users

A "one-stop shop" model is preferable where all the required services for physical and mental health and drug use are located together in the same setting. If this is not possible, it is important to have referral pathways and linkages to other local services.

Depending on the context, the alternatives for delivering PHCS include:

- Drop-in centres
- Community or general practice clinics
- Outpatient drug treatment centres
- Hospital-based PHCS
- Closed setting-based health services
- Community outreach and home-based care

DROP-IN CENTRES

Drop-in centres (DICs) are common throughout the world. They have been demonstrated to have a positive effect on increasing knowledge among DUs on HIV/AIDS prevention, overdose prevention and other health outcomes. A small health-care team, comprising doctors, nurses, health workers, peer educators or outreach workers can effectively deliver PHCS in DICs.

DICs provide a range of services such as peer support, information, education, needle-and-syringe programmes, referral and other health services (including OST and antiretroviral therapy [ART]), and social and recreational activities. Outreach services are an essential component of DICs. They target DUs and their partners.

DICs are places that DUs feel safe in, as they are less stigmatizing and more accessible to substance-using populations.

COMMUNITY OR GENERAL PRACTICE CLINICS

All clinic staff members should be trained to provide services in a non-judgemental and empathetic manner for DUs to continue accessing the service. Most community clinics in Asia have a nurse and/or a full or part-time doctor.

OUTPATIENT DRUG TREATMENT CENTRES

These provide on-site PHCS for DUs. They are co-located with an outpatient drug treatment programme and thus offer an ideal setting to implement directly observed treatment, short-course (DOTS) for TB or OST. They can also be used to provide ART to increase the adherence to treatment.

HOSPITAL-BASED PHCS

In many settings, DUs access hospital-based care particularly where community-based services are limited. Primary or emergency care medical and paramedical personnel should be trained in working with DUs, particularly in the management and prevention of overdose and other acute conditions. These settings offer an ideal opportunity for referral to other specialist services.

CLOSED SETTING-BASED HEALTH SERVICES FOR DUs

Prisons have large numbers of incarcerated DUs. Prison health services should provide prevention and treatment, as well as care services for DUs with HIV-related and other illnesses. These should include testing and counselling services for HIV, OST, DOTS for TB, management of opportunistic infections (OIs) and ART for DUs living with HIV.

Continuity of care is essential during the transition from closed settings to the community.

COMMUNITY OUTREACH AND HOME-BASED CARE

Community-level care includes DU networks; community-based care organizations (CBOs); nongovernmental organizations (NGOs); needle–syringe programmes; health posts staffed by community health workers or auxiliary nurses. Basic health care can be delivered through trained peer workers, outreach workers, community health workers and auxiliary nurses.

Community care is used to reach out to hidden DUs, recognize problems early (e.g. referring cases needing further attention) and follow up patients (e.g. ensuring adherence to HIV treatment). Where appropriate, family members should be involved by the PHCS staff in the treatment process.

1.7 Comprehensive service package for drug users[13,14]

This includes the following components:
- Provide care and support for HIV-positive DUs including ART.
- Provide services for the prevention, diagnosis and treatment of TB; and prevention and treatment of other OIs.

- Provide condoms, and clean needles and syringes (outreach workers can provide these).
- Screen for sexually transmitted infections (STI) and provide clinical services and treatment where indicated.
- Diagnose and treat viral hepatitis (hepatitis B and C) and provide vaccination for hepatitis B.
- Offer HIV testing and counselling.
- Provide OST and other drug dependency treatment.
- Provide targeted IEC for DUs and their sexual partners.

The package should include outreach services, which are very helpful in bringing hidden populations of DUs to care and treatment services, and increasing access. Outreach workers can also provide IEC. In addition, clients registered at the PHCS should be regularly followed up and referral support provided to clients for conditions that cannot be treated on site.

The guiding principles for establishing services for DUs and guidelines for minimum staff requirements, equipment, facilities and training necessary for the PHCS are provided in Annex 1.

Common health problems associated with drug use/injecting drug use 2

Table 1. Common health problems associated with drug use/ injecting drug use

Injection-related injuries and infections	
Injection-related injuries	• Bruising • Scarring • Swelling and inflammation including urticaria • Venous injury • Arterial injury • Ulcers
Injection-related infections	• Cellulitis and abscess • Thrombophlebitis
Complications of injection-related infections	• Bacteraemia and septicaemia • Musculoskeletal infections • Endovascular complications • Tetanus
Infectious diseases	
	• Sexually transmitted infections • Viral hepatitis (hepatitis B and C) • Respiratory tract infections • Tuberculosis (TB) • HIV/AIDS
Non-infectious disorders	
	• Psychiatric disorders • Substance dependence and substance use-related disorders
Other common health problems	
	• Pain • Constipation • Poor dental condition/hygiene

2.1 Injection-related injuries

2.1.1 Bruising

Bruising occurs when blood leaks out from the vein under the skin during the process of injecting. Bruising at the injection site can reflect poor injection techniques.

- ■ Prevention
- Education on safe injecting practices is helpful in preventing bruising, such as applying adequate pressure for a sufficient amount of time after injecting.
- Using a new needle for each injection and rotating the injecting sites can help in preventing bruising.
- Using a soft, flexible, easy-to-open tourniquet and removing it before injecting prevents bruising.

- ■ Treatment
- There is no specific treatment.
- Topical creams are not useful in treating bruising.

2.1.2 Scarring (track marks)

Track marks are scars along the veins caused by repeated injecting into the same site.

- ■ Prevention
- Alternating and rotating the injecting site will reduce scarring.
- Using a sharp, sterile needle for each injection will also reduce scarring.

- ■ Treatment
- There is no specific treatment.
- For keloids and heavy scarring, refer the DU to a specialist.

2.1.3 Swelling and inflammation including urticaria

Redness or swelling around the injection site may occur if the vein is missed and the drug is injected into the soft tissue. Urticaria is a "histamine reaction", a direct result of the drug entering the soft tissues.

- ■ Prevention
- Making sure that there is venous access before injecting prevents leakage into the soft tissues.

- ■ Treatment
- There is no specific treatment.
- Application of cold compresses initially and warm compresses later may be useful.
- It usually resolves without treatment in a few days.
- Urticaria is difficult to prevent but resolves without treatment.

2.1.4 Venous injury

Veins collapse is due to repeated injections at the same site. Other causes include repeated local infections leading to scarring of the vein; trauma to the vein and/or surrounding tissues; use of irritant substances; and using a barbed or blunt needle which tears the vein, damages the valves in the vein and leads to a large amount of scarring.

Chronic venous insufficiency occurs due to chronic damage to the veins. The walls of the veins and the valves get damaged so the blood cannot return to the heart as fast as it is pumped. Venous ulcers occur as a complication of venous stasis. Injection sites can have persistent ulcers.

- ■ Prevention
- Choosing a large vein for injecting, cleaning the site well with alcohol and putting pressure on the injection site after injecting for at least 30 seconds prevents vein injury.
- A vein collapse can be prevented by always alternating and rotating the injection site and by injecting in the direction of the body's blood flow.
- Inserting the needle at an angle of 15–45 degrees with the bevel of needle facing upwards is helpful.

■ Treatment
- Normal saline may be used on the wound and the part kept dry.
- Povidone solution can also be used.
- If the wound is large, dressings that encourage tissue growth and reduce infection should be used.

2.1.5 Arterial injury

Arterial injury results from inadvertent injection into the artery. This is more common when a vein is located close to an artery such as in the groin. Arterial injuries can result in haemorrhage.

The inadvertent injection of drugs into the arterial circulation can also result in vascular spasm with loss of distal tissue due to lack of blood flow. This may be complicated by infection (gas gangrene or tetanus) and muscle swelling (compartment syndrome), which may lead to amputation and renal failure.

■ Prevention
- A pulsating blood vessel should not be used for injection.
- Adequate pressure should be applied for at least 15 minutes if an artery is punctured or the drug is inadvertently injected intra-arterially.

■ Treatment
- If there is significant haemorrhage, refer the DU to a hospital.

2.2 Injection-related infections

Cellulitis is a bacterial infection of the skin resulting in the skin becoming red, hot, swollen and tender. Cellulitis and abscesses often occur together.

An **abscess** is a collection of pus under the skin. Many DUs who have been injecting for more than ten years develop chronic, recurrent abscesses that may be related to colonization with an abscess-inducing subspecies of a common skin bacterium (*Staphylococcus aureus*).

Thrombophlebitis is an infection of the vein wall. It can be an extension of cellulitis or due to an infected clot within the vein.

Common health problems associated with drug use/injecting drug use

- **Risk factors**
- Poor injection technique
- Injecting tablets (particularly diverted buprenorphine or dextropropoxyphene)
- Injecting frequently
- Injecting frequently at the same sites
- Using non-sterile injecting equipment
- Not cleaning the skin adequately before injecting
- Resorting to skin popping (experienced IDUs who do not have accessible/patent veins for injecting resort to "skin popping" – subcutaneous or intramuscular injection)
- Injecting "cocktails" (for example, mixtures of benzodiazepines, antihistamines and heroin or dextropropoxyphene)
- "Booting" (repeatedly flushing and pulling back during injection)
- Being HIV-positive
- Having a poor nutritional status.

- **Prevention**
- Maintaining skin hygiene and hand-washing
- Using clean injecting equipment every time
- Reducing the frequency of injections
- Ensuring early diagnosis and treatment.

- **Clinical features**
- Symptoms associated with cellulitis and abscesses take between 2 and 5 days to develop. The part may be hot, red, swollen, tender and fluctuant (indicating pus formation).
- Abscesses in the buttock area can continue to grow for many weeks without producing any symptoms, resulting in a cavity that may be filled with up to a litre of pus.
- Veins may show tenderness and swelling.

Assess to determine the following:
- Which wounds need referral to a hospital?

- Which wounds are true abscesses that need incision and drainage?
- Which wounds need conservative treatment such as antibiotics?
- Which wounds need antibiotics followed by incision and drainage?

■ Treatment

Cellulitis

Some abscesses present with an area of erythema that is beyond the boundaries of the abscess itself. These need to be monitored closely and treated with broad-spectrum antibiotics to prevent rapid progression (*see* Table 2).

Abscess
- If the abscess is fluctuant or if pus is found on aspiration, the recommended treatment is incision and drainage by a trained professional (referral to a hospital may be required).
- The wound should be cleaned with alcohol wipes followed by application of povidone solution to cover the wound and at least a three-inch margin around the site.
- Analgesia may be necessary.
- Primary-care providers should not perform incision and drainage above major arteries and near joints. Knowledge of normal human anatomy is an important prerequisite for performing incision and drainage.
- Irrigating the wound with sterile saline can be useful in large and complex wounds.
- Following drainage, the wound should be covered with a bulky gauze dressing to absorb the continued discharge of serosanguineous fluid.
- The packing should be changed every other day and the wound inspected to ascertain whether the skin has broken down or erythema is progressing.

Refer to Annex 4 for sample educational material on reducing the occurrence of abscess and cellulitis.

Thrombophlebitis
- Bed rest for prolonged periods should be avoided. It can make the symptoms worse.

- Ibuprofen, an anti-inflammatory medication, may help lessen the pain and inflammation.
- Prescription leg compression stockings (knee or thigh high) improve blood flow and may help to relieve pain and swelling.
- Antibiotics may be required if there is fever or obvious signs of infection.
- If the infection has spread to the deep veins, anticoagulants may be needed.

Antibiotics are usually unnecessary for the treatment of abscesses following incision and drainage. In the context of associated cellulitis, an antibiotic (e.g. cloxacillin) is recommended following successful incision and drainage.

Table 2. Antibiotic treatment of injection-related injury

Body weight (in kg)	Medication
<50	CLOXACILLIN (tablet) Give 250 mg orally 4 times daily for 5 days
>50	500 mg x 4 times/day for 5 days **OR**
	CEFIXIME (tablet) 400 mg/day in two divided doses for 5–7 days

Table 3. Antibiotic treatment of severe injection-related injury

Weight (in kg)	CLOXACILLIN (injection) Dose: 25–50 mg/kg
	Intravenous (IV): To a vial of 500 mg add 8 ml of sterile water to give 500 mg/10 ml Intramuscular (IM): Add 1.3 ml of sterile water to a vial of 250 mg to give 250 mg/1.5 ml
30–39	6–12 ml IM (20–40 ml IV)
40–49	7.5–15 ml IM (25–50 ml IV)
50–59	9–18 ml IM (30–60 ml IV)
60–69	10–20 ml IM (35–70 ml IV)
	If not able to refer: Give above dose IV/IM every 4–6 hours

For severe cellulitis refractory to cloxacillin or cefixime, switch to ceftriaxone.

Table 4. Antibiotic treatment of complicated injection-related injury

Body weight (in kg)	CEFTRIAXONE* (vial)
<50	50–100 mg per kg body weight per day IM or IV for 7–14 days
>50	1–2 g/day IM or IV for 7–14 days

* Ceftriaxone should be administered at the same time each day to maintain blood levels of the drug.

■ Follow-up care

Patients should return to have the wound checked within 24 hours following incision and drainage. Following this the wound should be reviewed regularly to ensure it has healed without complication. If antibiotics have been prescribed, patients should be instructed to complete the full course of medications to reduce the likelihood of development of drug-resistant bacteria. Analgesia may be required if pain persists. Anticoagulants may be required for thrombophlebitis if it has spread to the deep veins.

■ Complications

- Bacteraemia and septicaemia, with the formation of multiple new abscesses ("seeding" of infection) such as in the joints, pleura or other areas
- Gangrene (tissue death): darkening of the affected tissue; pungent odour; loss of sensation

> **PRACTICAL POINTS**
> - Education on safe injecting practices, which includes the use of clean needles and syringes, is essential in preventing injection-related harm and infections.
> - While many abscesses can be treated with simple incision and drainage, in rare cases there may be complications that can lead to sepsis, amputation and death.
> - It is estimated that one out of every three IDUs has an active abscess at any given time.
> - Clinical examination is critical as DUs may not complain of pain.
> - OST is one of the most effective interventions to reduce the likelihood of developing injection-related infections among opioid injectors.

2.3 Complications of injection-related infections

2.3.1 Bacteraemia and septicaemia

Bacteraemia is the presence of bacteria in the bloodstream.
- It is a common complication of injecting drug use.
- It is mainly caused by the insertion of skin flora into the vascular system.
- Poverty, poor nutrition, poor dental hygiene/condition, leg ulcers may contribute to bacteraemia.

Bacteraemia can lead to complications such as septicaemia which can result in endocarditis and septic embolism, musculoskeletal infections and tetanus of the wound.

Septicaemia is an established blood infection resulting from bacteraemia.

■ Risk factors
- Untreated injection-related infections
- Other untreated infections such as dental abscesses, ulcers

■ Prevention
- Treat the source of infection (*see* Tables 2, 3 and 4).

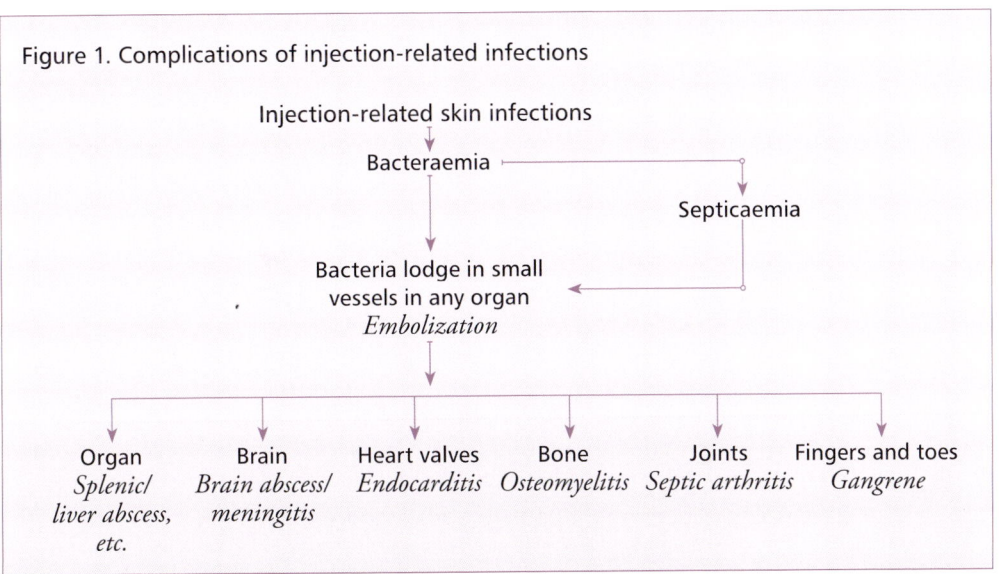

Figure 1. Complications of injection-related infections

- **Clinical features**
- Initial symptoms include high fever (>38.5ºC) with chills and rigors, vomiting and exhaustion.
- Physical signs include tachycardia, hypotension and delirium.
- This may progress to altered consciousness, confusion and even seizures in severe sepsis.

- **Treatment**
- Refer the patient immediately to hospital.
- Give the patient bed rest.
- Provide initial supportive measures including oxygen and IV fluids. Insert an IV line before referring the patient (if an intact vein is available).
- If possible, consider drawing blood for culture prior to starting appropriate IV/IM antibiotics.
  First-line therapy includes cloxacillin plus gentamicin (*see* Table 5):
  – Alternative: ampicillin plus gentamicin (ampicillin 1 g vial x 3, gentamicin 1.5 ml of a 160 mg ampoule x 2; duration dependent on severity. Change to oral ampicillin as soon as possible).
  Second-line therapy: ceftriaxone: 1–2 g once daily
  – By deep IM injection (if dose=2 g then inject 1 g into each buttock; mix with lignocaine to reduce pain)
  – By slow IV (over 3 minutes)
  – By infusion (over 30 minutes)

- **Prognosis**
- Septicaemia can be fatal.

> **PRACTICAL POINT**
> To prevent septicaemia, everything that is used during the injecting process must be clean (swabbing the spoon used for dissolving the drugs, using clean sterile water and swabbing the arm before injecting). Hand-washing should be encouraged as a normal part of injecting.

Table 5. Antibiotic treatment of injection-related bacterial septicaemia

Weight (in kg)	Cloxacillin Dose: 25–50 mg/kg	Gentamicin Dose: 5 mg/kg/day Calculate exact dose based on body weight. Use these doses only if this is not possible.	
	IV: To a vial of 500 mg add 8 ml of sterile water to give 500 mg/10 ml OR IM*: Add 1.3 ml of sterile water to a vial of 250 mg to give 250 mg/1.5 ml	Vial containing 20 mg = 2 ml (10 mg/ml undiluted)	Vial containing 80 mg = 2 ml (40 mg/ml undiluted)
30–39	6–12 ml IM* (20–40 ml IV)	15–19 ml IM*/IV	4–5 ml IM*/IV
40–49	7.5–15 ml IM* (25–50 ml IV)	20–24 ml IM*/IV	5–6 ml IM*/IV
50–59	9–18 ml IM* (30–60 ml IV)	25–29 ml IM*/IV	6–7 ml IM*/IV
60–69	10–20 ml IM* (35–70 ml IV)	30–34 ml IM*/IV	7.5–8.6 ml IM*/IV
	If not able to refer: Give above dose IV/IM* every 4–6 hours	If not able to refer: Give above dose once daily	

*IM if there is difficulty in accessing a vein in IDUs

2.3.2 Thrombosis

Injecting drug use is generally associated with clot formation in the veins that are frequently used for injecting. Chronic venous damage or infection of the skin tissues or veins is considered a risk factor for the development of deep vein thrombosis.

The repeated trauma of venepuncture, local infections and the irritant properties of the injected substance are the main causes of superficial and deep venous thrombosis.

Septic thrombosis is responsible for bacteraemia and can lead to the other complications discussed earlier. High-risk locations for the development of complicating embolization include deep venous thrombosis of the iliofemoral and upper limb veins.

■ Risk factors and prevention
- Repeated venepuncture leading to damage of the veins
- Unwashed skin
- Using unsterile injecting equipment
- Injecting irritant substances
- Pre-existing infections such as cellulitis and abscesses. These conditions must be promptly treated to prevent spread and the formation of clots in the vein.

■ Clinical features
- There is usually a slow onset of a tender red area along the superficial veins of the skin. A long, thin red area may be seen as the inflammation follows the path of a superficial vein.
- This area may feel hard, warm and tender. The skin around the vein may be itchy, tender and swollen.
- The area may begin to throb or burn.
- Symptoms may be worse when the leg is lowered, especially when first getting out of bed in the morning.
- A low-grade fever may occur.
- If an infection is present, symptoms may include redness, fever, pain, swelling, or breakdown of the skin.

2.3.2.1 Deep vein thrombosis
- This can be similar in presentation to superficial phlebitis, but some people may have no symptoms.
- The classical signs and symptoms include redness, warmth, swelling and pain in the leg.
- There may be pain and swelling throughout the entire limb. For example, one side of the lower leg may swell for no apparent reason.

■ **Treatment**
- Bed rest for prolonged periods should be avoided.
- Deep vein thrombosis requires immediate care and hospitalization.
- Ultrasonography can be used to detect the presence of clots in the veins.
- Ibuprofen, an anti-inflammatory medication, may help lessen the pain and inflammation.
- Prescription leg compression stockings (knee or thigh high) improve blood flow and may help to relieve pain and swelling.
- Antibiotics should be given (*see* Table 5).
- Anticoagulants should be started and continued for at least 3–6 months. An injectable anticoagulant such as enoxaparin is started initially along with warfarin, an oral drug which takes time to reach effective levels for anticoagulation*.

2.3.2.2 Embolism

An embolism is the passage of particles (such as blood clots, bacteria or undissolved injected drug) through the bloodstream. It can be due to an infected blood clot getting dislodged from a vein following thrombosis. Emboli can lodge in the small vessels of any organ causing tissue damage and infection. Examples include stroke (brain) and gangrene of the fingers and toes (*see* Figure 1).

■ **Risk factors**
- Thrombosis of the veins
- Crushing and injecting tablets
- Septicaemia

■ **Prevention**
- Advise against crushing and injecting crushed pills.
- Advise that the drug to be injected should be adequately dissolved.
- Suggest the use of a filter to catch large particles during preparation of the injection.
- Endovascular clots should be treated promptly.

---

*The use of warfarin requires ongoing monitoring of the international normalized ratio (INR). Adherence to the regimen must be ensured. Patients must be cautioned to report for blood tests as advised.

■ Clinical features
These would depend on the site where the embolus is lodged. An embolus can be life-threatening. Examples include the following:
- Chest pain and shortness of breath (embolus in the lung)
- Hemiparesis or hemiplegia (embolus in the brain, also known as stroke)
- Sudden loss of vision, speech (embolus in the blood vessels of the eye or speech area of the brain)
- Gangrene of the fingers and toes (embolus in the distal blood vessels)
- Organ abscesses (emboli in various organs such as the spleen, joints)

■ Treatment
- Give symptomatic treatment with analgesics, oxygen, bed rest.
- Start anticoagulants.
- Specific treatment depends on the site of embolization.

2.3.3 Musculoskeletal infections
The common musculoskeletal infections that complicate injection-related infections are:
- Septic arthritis
- Osteomyelitis
- Gangrene.

■ Risk factors
- Local extension of a skin or soft tissue infection and spread of bacteria

■ Prevention
- Treat the source of infection (*see* Tables 3 and 4).

■ Clinical features
- The usual sites of infection are muscles and joints adjacent to injection sites; the spine and knee.
- Unusual sites of infection are the sternoclavicular and sacroiliac joints.
- Infections may be indolent, and the only symptom may be pain without fever.

- Septic arthritis: there is inability to move the joints and they may be swollen and painful.
- Osteomyelitis: suspect osteomyelitis if the abscess or cellulitis is close to a bony structure; it causes deep-seated pain.
- Gangrene: there is darkening of the affected tissue; pungent odour; loss of sensation.

■ Treatment

Septic arthritis, osteomyelitis
- Ensure rest to the affected joint.
- Manage pain (*see* section 2.6.1).
- Give IV or IM antibiotics.
    – *First-line:* cloxacillin IV or IM (*see* Table 5)
    – *Alternative regimen:* ampicillin and gentamicin (slow IV/IM/infusion
    – ampicillin 1–2 g every 6 hours; gentamicin 5 mg/kg/day)
- Referral is required for further investigations (e.g. X-ray or culture) and treatment.
- Arthrocentesis may be done, if needed.

Gangrene
- Gangrene is death of tissue (necrosis). It is a serious condition that requires prompt surgical care.

■ Prognosis
- The immediate prognosis for IDUs with skeletal infection is good with appropriate treatment.

2.3.4 Endovascular complications
Endovascular infections in IDUs include:
- Infective endocarditis
- Organ abscesses (brain and liver abscess)
- Mycotic aneurysms

2.3.4.1 Infective endocarditis
- The estimated incidence is 1.5–3.3 cases per 1000 IDUs per year.[15]
- The commonest causative organism is *Staphylococcus aureus.*
- The tricuspid valve is often involved in IDUs.

■ **Risk factors**
- Infection at other sites
- A past history of infective endocarditis
- A past history of rheumatic heart disease
- High frequency of injecting and unsafe injecting
- HIV infection

■ **Clinical features**
- There may be fever, dyspnoea, pleuritic chest pain and cough.
- A murmur may be absent.
- Complications such as brain and splenic abscesses may occur owing to septic embolization.

■ **Treatment**
- First-line treatment is with IV administration of cloxacillin plus gentamicin (*see* Table 5) for at least 4 weeks. Ampicillin plus gentamicin is also given (ampicillin 1 g vial x 3, gentamicin 1.5 ml of 160 mg ampoule x 2; duration dependent on severity. Change to oral ampicillin as soon as possible).
- Severe endocarditis or endocarditis with complications may require 6 weeks or more of therapy.
- If left untreated, infective endocarditis has a high mortality rate.

2.3.4.2 Organ abscess
An organ abscess is a serious infection which generally requires hospital care. Symptoms depend on the organ affected.

2.3.4.3 Mycotic aneurysms
A mycotic aneurysm is an infected aneurysm, generally in the arterial circulation. It is a serious condition that requires prompt surgical care and antibiotics.

Refer to Annex 3 for a comprehensive table on antibiotics used to treat injection-related infections and their complications.

2.3.5 Tetanus

Tetanus is an infection caused by *Clostridium tetani*. Drug injection provides several potential sources for infection with *C. tetani*, including the drug itself, its adulterants, injection equipment and unwashed skin. Although recommendations to prevent transmission of HIV among IDUs may limit infection from contaminated injection equipment, these measures may not be effective against spores inoculated from the skin or contained in the drug. Therefore, prevention efforts should emphasize vaccination for tetanus.[16]

■ Clinical features

Tetanus occurs in communities that do not have a routine tetanus vaccination programme. It causes muscle spasm which can lead to death if the muscles of respiration are affected.

■ Prevention
- Tetanus is almost entirely preventable through vaccination and appropriate wound care.
- Check the tetanus toxoid (TT) immunization status at routine clinic visits:
  – When was TT last given?
  – Which dose of TT was this?

If tetanus toxoid is due:
• Give 0.5 ml IM in the upper arm after cleaning the skin with an alcohol swab. • Advise when the next dose is due. • Keep a record.

Tetanus toxoid (TT) schedule	
• At first contact	TT1
• At least four weeks after TT1	TT2
• At least six months after TT2	TT3
• At least one year after TT3	TT4
• At least one year after TT4	TT5

2.4 Infectious diseases

2.4.1 Sexually transmitted infections (STIs)

2.4.1.1 Overlapping risks
- High rates of STIs are seen among DUs.
- STIs have been shown to be independent risk factors for the sexual transmission of HIV.
- DUs frequently trade sex for drugs and therefore have a higher risk of acquiring STIs including HIV.
- DUs taking ATS may indulge in frequent high-risk (unprotected) sexual activity and therefore their chances for acquiring STI including HIV are greater.

■ Prevention
- Correct and consistent use of condoms
- Regular testing for STIs including HIV (including partner/s where possible)
- Early treatment if symptoms present
- Good genital hygiene (including partner)

2.4.1.2 Syndromic management of STIs
Primary health-care facilities in resource-constrained countries lack the equipment and trained personnel required to make an aetiological diagnosis of STIs. To overcome this problem, a syndrome-based approach to the management of STI patients has been developed and promoted by WHO.[17] The syndromic approach can be followed by an aetiological diagnosis if diagnostic facilities are available.

2.4.1.3 Diagnosis of STIs using the syndromic approach
■ History-taking
- The clinician should ask substance users about symptoms of STIs, and sexual risk behaviours.
  STI syndromes
  – Male urethral discharge and/or dysuria

- Genital ulcer disease (GUD)
- Inguinal bubo
- Scrotal swelling
- Abnormal vaginal discharge
- Lower abdominal pain in sexually active women

Sexual risk behaviours
- Unsafe sex – no or inconsistent condom use
- Commercial sex work and exchanging sex for drugs or money
- Multiple sex partners (male and female) or concurrent sex partners
- ATS use and increased levels of unsafe sex
- Alcohol use before and during sex, and practising unsafe sex

■ Clinical features

The following questions may guide the syndromic management of STIs in DUs and their partners (Table 6).

Table 6. History-taking for the syndromic management of sexually transmitted infections

Questions related to STIs	Syndromes
Is there vaginal discharge that is abnormal in colour, odour, amount or consistency? Do you have itching or irritation of the vulva or vagina? Do you have pain during urination?	Abnormal vaginal discharge
Do you have pain in the lower abdomen? Do you have pain during sexual intercourse?	Lower abdominal pain
Is there a discharge from the urethra? Do you have pain during urination?	Urethral discharge
Is there any ulcer, sore or blister on your genitalia? Do you have discharge, sores or warts in and around the anus? Are there ulcers and other lesions in and around the mouth?	Genital ulcer
Do you have any of the following: swelling, lumps or ulcers in the groin area?	Inguinal bubo

■ Education and counselling for STIs
- Education and counselling for DUs should be done in private, confidential settings.
- Educate DUs that most STIs can be cured, except HIV, herpes and genital warts.
- Sex with an untreated partner can lead to reinfection. Treatment of the partner, even if they have no symptoms, is important for the health of the partner and the DU/IDU.
- Promote safer sexual behaviours to prevent HIV and STIs.
  – Counsel on safer sex (sexual activity to be limited during treatment).
  – Counsel on consistent condom use with all partners.
- Emphasize compliance with treatment.
- Examine barriers to prevention, discuss solutions and build skills for safer sex.
- Advise on HIV testing and counselling.
- Partner notification: The care provider should strongly encourage the regular sex partners of DUs to attend the primary health-care facility to check for STIs and offer education and counselling about the prevention, early diagnosis and treatment of STIs.

Presumptive treatment of sex workers with risk criteria (exposure to unprotected sex) and sexual partners of DUs with STIs is recommended. Refer to the national guidelines for the treatment of STIs.

> **PRACTICAL POINTS**
>
> The **syndromic management of STIs** is based on the identification of consistent groups of symptoms and easily recognized signs (syndromes), and the provision of treatment that will deal with the majority of, or the most serious, organisms responsible for producing a syndrome.
>
> Where/whenever possible, it is recommended to use single-dose therapy for the treatment of STI.

Figure 2. Management of urethral discharge/dysuria without microscopy

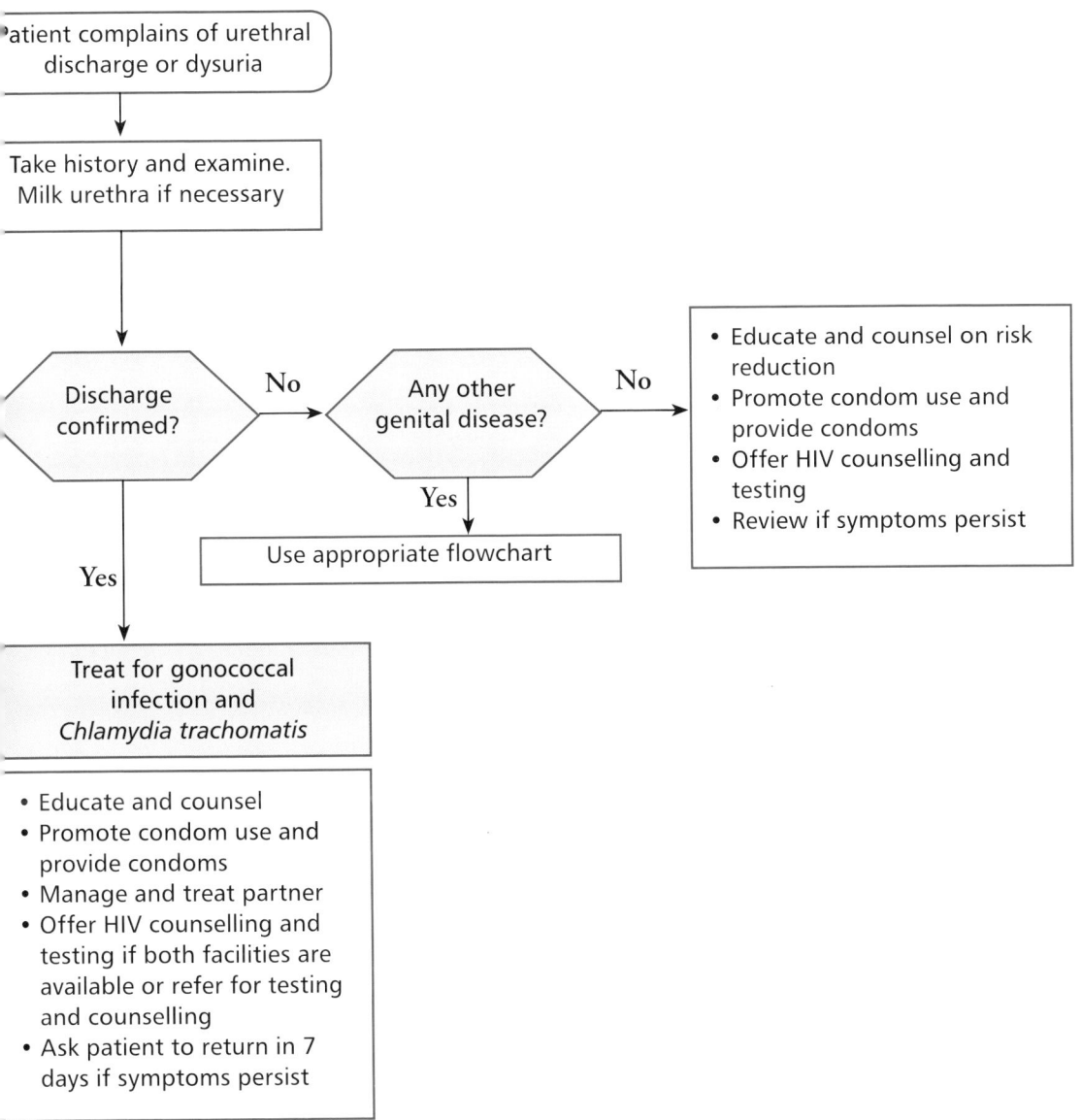

Source: *Regional guidelines for the management of sexually transmitted infections.* New Delhi, WHO Regional Office for South-East Asia, 2007 (draft).[18]

Figure 3. Management of abnormal vaginal discharge

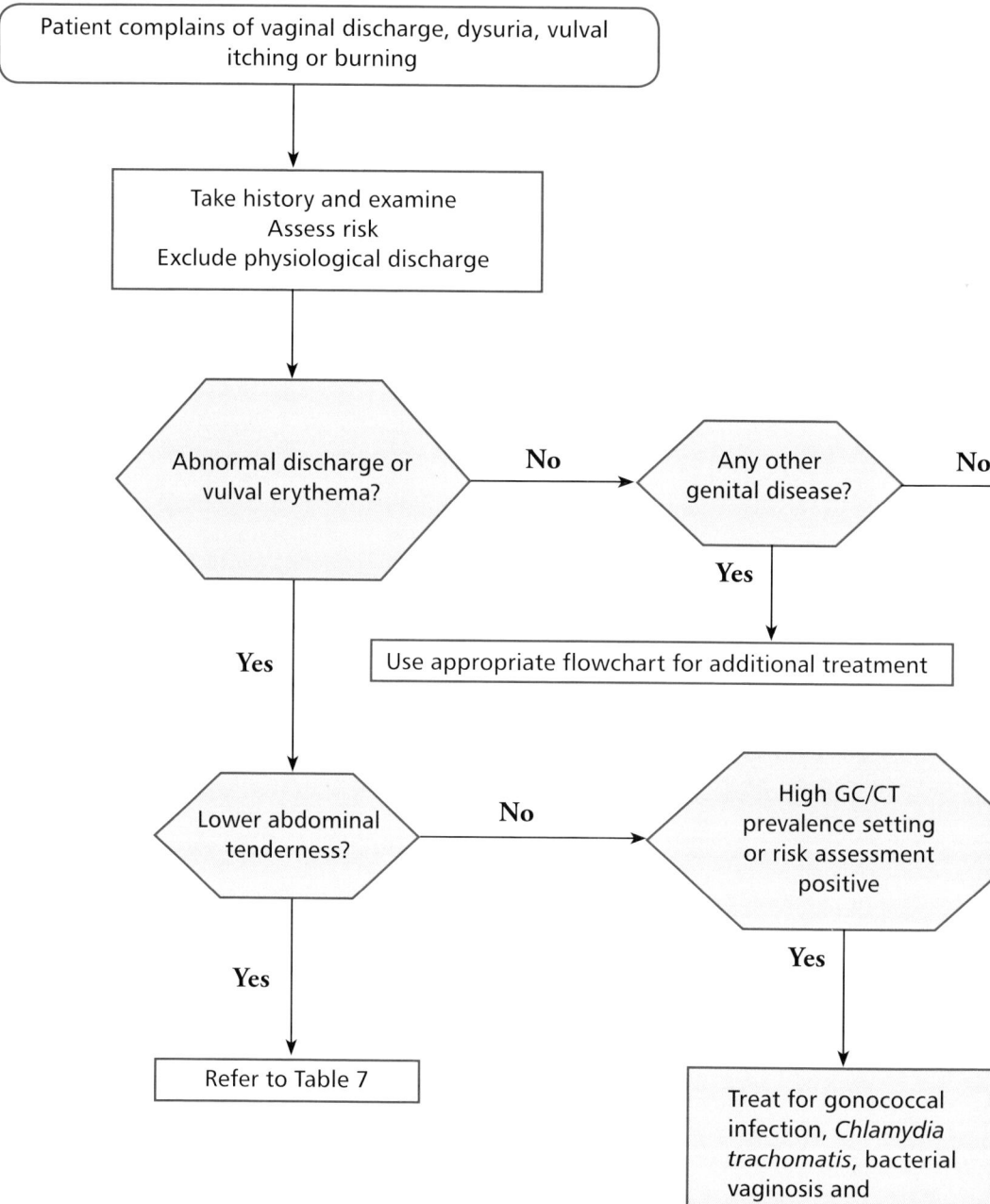

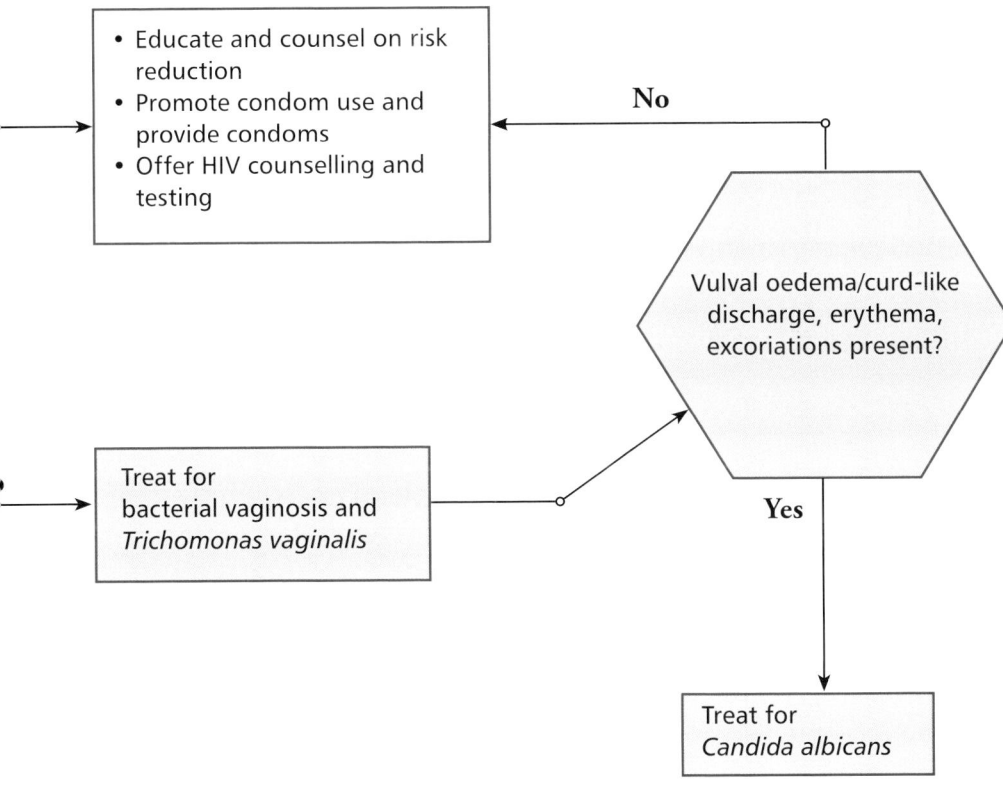

Source: *Regional guidelines for the management of sexually transmitted infections.* New Delhi, WHO Regional Office for South-East Asia, 2007 (draft).[18]

GC/CT: gonococcal infection/*Chlamydia trachomatis*

Management of common health problems of drug users

Figure 4. Management of genital ulcers

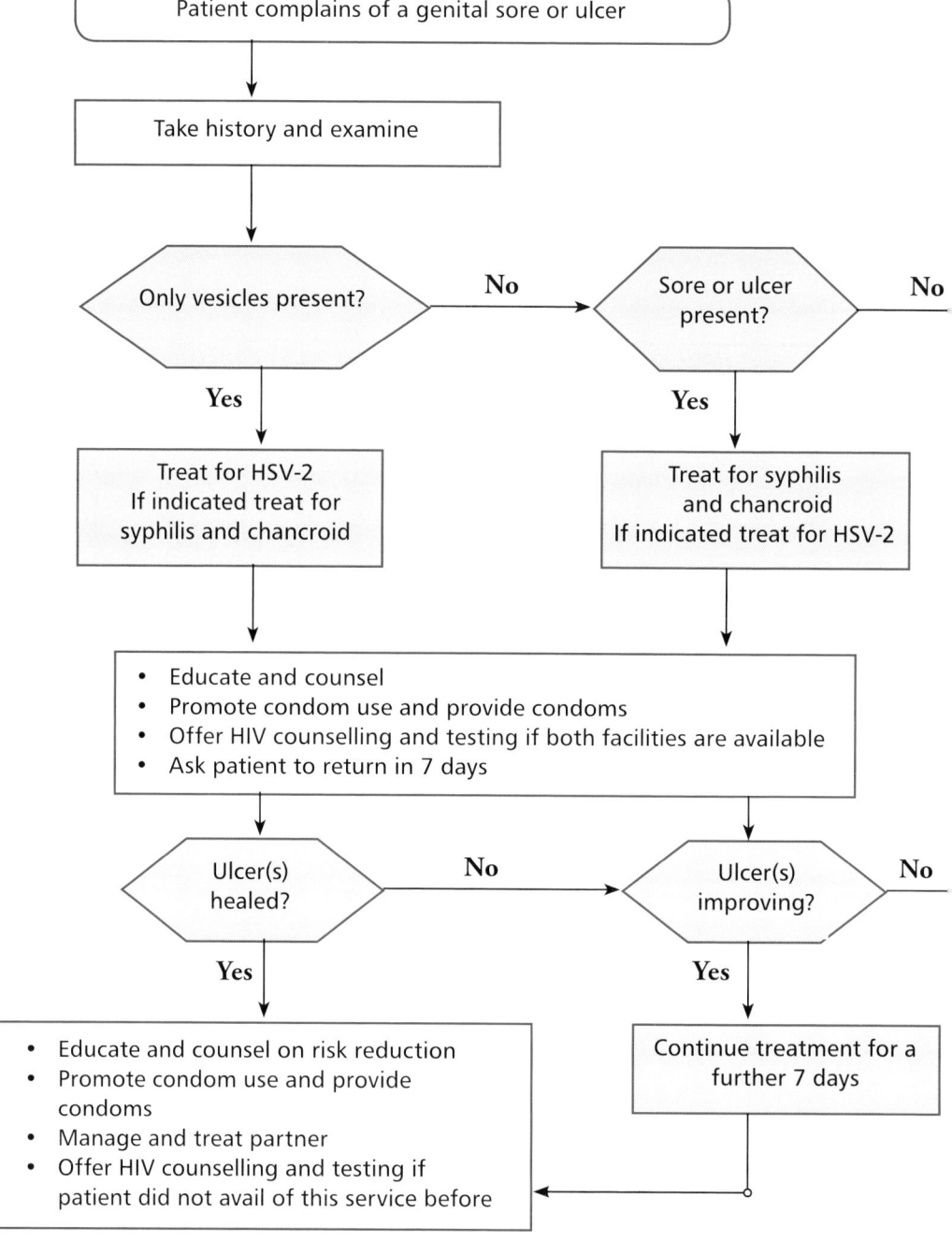

Common health problems associated with drug use/injecting drug use

→
- Educate and counsel
- Promote condom use and provide condoms
- Offer HIV counselling and testing
- Review in 7 days

→ Refer

Source: *Regional guidelines for the management of sexually transmitted infections.* New Delhi, WHO Regional Office for South-East Asia, 2007 (draft).[18]

2.4.1.4 Management of sexually transmitted infections

Table 7 provides information on the syndromic management of STIs.

Table 7. Syndromic management of sexually transmitted infections

Syndrome	Disease	Drug
Urethral discharge (men) **Note**: Patients should be advised to return if symptoms persist after 7 days of therapy.	Treat **gonorrhoea** **PLUS** **chlamydial infection**	cefixime 400 mg orally as a single dose OR ceftriaxone 125 mg by IM injection as a single dose OR spectinomycin 2 g by IM injection as a single dose **PLUS** azithromycin 1 g orally, in a single dose OR doxycycline[2] 100 mg orally twice daily for 7 days OR tetracycline, 500 mg orally, 4 times a day for 7 days
Abnormal vaginal discharge (women) and cervical infection	Treat **bacterial vaginosis** **PLUS** **trichomoniasis** **PLUS** Symptoms consistent with **candidiasis**	metronidazole[1] 2 g orally as a single dose OR metronidazole[1] 400–500 mg orally twice daily for 7 days **PLUS** clotrimazole 500 mg intravaginally as a single dose OR nystatin 100 000 IU intravaginally once daily for 14 days OR miconazole or clotrimazole 200 mg intravaginally once daily for 3 days

Syndrome	Disease	Drug
Genital ulcer disease (men and women)	Treat **syphilis**	Benzathine penicillin G 2.4 million IU, by IM injection at a single session (split into 2 doses at separate sites) OR tetracycline[2] 500 mg orally 4 times daily for 15 days OR doxycycline[2] 100 mg orally twice daily for 15 days OR erythromycin 500 mg orally 4 times daily for 15 days
	PLUS	**PLUS**
	chancroid	azithromycin 1 g orally as a single dose OR erythromycin 500 mg orally 3 times daily for 7 days OR ciprofloxacin[1] 500 mg orally twice daily for 3 days
	PLUS	**PLUS**
	Symptoms consistent with **vesicles**	Where clinically indicated, acyclovir
	herpes simplex virus (HSV-2)	Primary infection: 200 mg five times daily for 7 days or 400 mg three times daily for 7 days Recurrent infection: As above except duration 5 days

Table 7 (*contd*). Syndromic management of sexually transmitted infections

Syndrome	Disease	Drug
Inguinal bubo without ulcer (men and women)	Treat **Lymphogranuloma venereum (LGV)**	doxycycline[2] 100 mg orally twice daily for 14 days OR tetracycline[2] 500 mg orally 4 times daily for 14 days OR erythromycin 500 mg orally daily for 14 days *Note* Some cases may require longer treatment than 14 days. Fluctuant lymph nodes should be aspirated through healthy skin. Incision and drainage or excision of nodes may delay healing and should not be attempted. Where there is doubt and/or treatment failure, referral for diagnostic biopsy is advisable.
Lower abdominal pain (women)	**Pelvic inflammatory disease (PID)**	ceftriaxone 250 mg by IM injection, as a single dose OR cefixime 400 mg orally as a single dose OR spectinomycin 2 g by IM injection as a single dose **PLUS** doxycycline 100 mg 2 times daily for 14 days **PLUS** metronidazole[1] 500 mg three times daily for 14 days

Syndrome	Disease	Drug
Warts (women, men)	**Genital warts**	Podophyllotoxin[2] 0.5% solution or gel twice daily for 3 days, followed by 4 days of no treatment, the cycle repeated up to 4 times (total volume of podophyllotoxin should not exceed 0.5 ml per day)

[1] Alcohol should be avoided while taking metronidazole to avoid a "disulfiram-type" reaction.
[2] Doxycycline, tetracycline and podophyllotoxin should not be used in pregnancy and during lactation.

2.4.1.5 Preventing STIs

Primary health-care team members play an important role in reinforcing behavioural risk-reduction measures. Counselling for consistent condom use and provision of condoms should be routine.

For further information please consult *Guidelines for the management of sexually transmitted infections* (WHO, 2003) and *Sexually transmitted and other reproductive tract infections: a guide to essential practice* (WHO, 2005).[17,19]

2.4.2 Viral hepatitis

An estimated 400 million persons worldwide are carriers of the hepatitis B virus (HBV).[20] Around 170 million individuals currently live with the hepatitis C virus (HCV).[20,21] HBV and HCV infections are very common among IDUs.

DUs are at high risk for infection with the hepatitis viruses, particularly HCV and HBV. Coinfection with HBV/HCV is common in the context of HIV among DUs.

- **Risk factors**
- Hepatitis B and C are transmitted by:
  - Contaminated blood and blood products
  - Sharing of contaminated injecting equipment including needles, syringes, spoons, filters
  - Needle-stick injuries in health-care settings

- Tattoos or piercing with contaminated equipment
- Sharing of razors and toothbrushes in closed settings (HBV)
- Mother-to-child transmission (MTCT) during pregnancy and delivery
- Unprotected sex (HBV)
• HCV is only rarely transmitted by the sexual route and usually only in the context of HCV/HIV coinfection.
• HCV is easily transmitted among individuals sharing injecting equipment.

Refer to Annex 4 for sample educational material on hepatitis B and C.

■ Clinical features of viral hepatitis
Acute infection
• Infection with HBV and HCV in early childhood is usually asymptomatic.
• 50–70% of adults experience symptoms during the acute phase of hepatitis B.
• <25% of adults experience symptoms in the acute phase of hepatitis C.
• Common symptoms are:
  - jaundice (HBV>HCV)
  - loss of appetite
  - upper abdominal pain
  - nausea
  - joint and muscle aches
  - dark-coloured urine and light-coloured stools (HBV>HCV)
  - lethargy and fatigue.

Chronic infection
Chronic infection is usually asymptomatic, or there may be non-specific symptoms such as fatigue and lethargy. Complications of chronic viral hepatitis include cirrhosis and hepatocellular carcinoma.

Acute episodes of hepatitis including fulminant hepatitis can occur in those with chronic hepatitis B in the context of acute hepatic injury from certain medications (e.g. ART) and alcohol.

The most important determinant of chronic infection with HBV is age. Most children who acquire the virus during the perinatal period will go on to develop chronic infection. Only a small proportion of adults with acute HBV go on to have chronic hepatitis B infection. Recovery from HBV infection is characterized by clearance of the hepatitis B surface antigen (HBsAg) and hepatitis B e antigen (HBeAg) from the blood following the development of antibodies to both antigens.

Three quarters of individuals with acute HCV infection go on to develop chronic hepatitis C regardless of age. In people infected only with hepatitis C, 5–15% will have liver-related complications such as cirrhosis or hepatocellular cancer. These complications develop over 10–40 years, depending on other comorbidities.

2.4.2.1 Viral hepatitis and HIV coinfection

Coinfection with HCV or HBV and HIV is relatively frequent, given the common routes of transmission.

The prevalence of chronic HBV infection in HIV-positive IDUs is usually the same as the general population, at around 10%. At least 75% of IDUs have been exposed to HBV in the past, though most clear the infection. The prevalence of chronic HCV infection in HIV-positive IDUs is usually >90%. The major risk in HBV/HIV coinfection is the immune reconstitution inflammatory syndrome (IRIS) following ART initiation, particularly in those with a low CD4 count.

HBV does not affect the progression of HIV, just as HIV does not affect the progression of HBV. HCV does not appear to dramatically affect the progression of HIV although some people with hepatitis C have a smaller increase in CD4 count on ART than those without it. HIV accelerates the progression of HCV, although with effective ART, the rate of progression is reduced. In HCV/HIV coinfection, there is a greater risk of developing some of the metabolic disorders that can be a side-effect of ART, such as insulin resistance and diabetes mellitus.

2.4.2.2 Management of viral hepatitis

■ Prevention

HBV vaccination is recommended for IDUs and health-care workers. The decision to recommend systematic vaccination for all should be made according to the prevalence of antibody to hepatitis B surface antigen (HBsAb) in a country. A pragmatic and opportunistic approach to hepatitis B vaccination is recommended in IDUs. Due to chaotic lifestyles, accelerated schedules are the most appropriate for this population. Pre-vaccination testing for hepatitis B is not necessary, and where testing is done, the first dose of the vaccination should be given at the same time.

Table 8. Schedule for hepatitis B vaccination

Vaccine	Age	Dose	Volume	No. of doses	Schedule
Engerix-B	<20 years	10 µg	0.5 ml	3	0, 1–2, 4 months†
	≥20 years	20 µg	1 ml	3	0, 1, 6 months†
Recombivax HB	≥20 years	10 µg	1 ml	3	0, 1, 6 months

Double-dose regimen is recommended in the context of HIV infection.
† An accelerated vaccination schedule of 0, 7 and 21 days for IDUs is sometimes recommended. This should be boosted at 1 year.
There is no vaccine for hepatitis C.

■ Treatment

General measures

Assess current alcohol use before initiating treatment and treat if necessary. It is recommended that no more than 10 g ethanol equivalents (standard drinks) be consumed per day.

People with hepatitis C and B are at increased risk for drug-induced liver toxicity by drugs such as ARVs (nevirapine, ritonavir, saquinavir, protease inhibitors), antituberculosis drugs (rifampicin, isoniazid), some analgesics (acetaminophen, diclofenac), antibiotics (ciprofloxacin, erythromycin), antifungal drugs (ketoconazole, fluconazole), valproic acid, statins, methyldopa, chlorpromazine, amiodarone, oral contraceptives.

Treatment of acute hepatitis
- Treatment for acute hepatitis B is aimed at symptomatic relief.
- Acute hepatitis C is rarely clinically apparent and therefore treatment is rarely needed. Symptomatic relief may be needed in a minority of cases. Although treatment of acute hepatitis C is available in some countries (interferon-based therapy), it is not yet widely available in the Region.

Treatment of chronic hepatitis
- Refer to a specialist for HBV and HCV treatment if significant liver enzyme abnormalities are present. A suggested level is 2.5 times normal, though treatment can be indicated even in the presence of normal liver function.
- Management of chronic hepatitis B requires the availability of testing for HBsAg, HBeAg and HBV DNA, while chronic hepatitis C treatment requires testing for viral HCV RNA.

Hepatitis B treatment consists of therapy with lamivudine (3TC), tenofovir (TDF), adefovir or pegylated interferon (PEG-IFN). Combination therapy may be indicated in some cases. Successful therapy results in the development of HBeAb or loss of HBeAg or HBV DNA.

Hepatitis C treatment consists of combination PEG-IFN and ribavirin therapy for 24–48 weeks depending on the HCV genotype. Side-effects can be significant, hence the need for specialist management.

Treatment of hepatitis and HIV coinfection
For patients coinfected with HIV and hepatitis B or C requiring treatment for only HIV or both hepatitis and HIV, medication decisions are based on recognition of the dual effect of some ARV drugs on HBV and HIV, such as 3TC and TDF.

HIV testing and counselling is recommended before treatment of hepatitis B and C, as this may complicate the treatment of HIV.

The best time to initiate HCV treatment is before ART is clinically indicated, as interactions with ART can be avoided and toxicity may be more easily managed. Hepatitis C treatment is more effective when the CD4 count is >350 cells/mm³.²²

2.4.2.3 Special considerations for HIV/HBV and HIV/HCV coinfection

Following initiation of ART in those with chronic HBV/HIV coinfection, immune reconstitution inflammatory syndrome (IRIS) from a hepatitis B flare can occur. It is more common in the presence of a low CD4 count. Refer to section 2.4.5.4 for further details.

The use of ARVs for the treatment of HIV with activity against HBV (such as 3TC or TDF) can reduce the progression of HBV in HBV/HIV coinfection.

Efficient HCV treatment, where possible, will facilitate the subsequent management with ART.

ART can be used safely and effectively in those coinfected with HIV and HCV. Initiation of ART in HCV/HIV coinfected patients should follow the current recommendations for HIV-monoinfected patients, with the exception that nevirapine (NVP) be avoided if possible and liver function tests are monitored closely. The choice of ART in HIV/HCV coinfection is determined by: the hepatotoxicity of some ART drugs (NVP); adherence (once-daily doses); drug interaction (zidovudine [ZDV] with ribavirin [RBV]); and coexisting psychiatric disorders such as depression. For example, hepatitis C treatment and efavirenz (EFV) can cause severe depression (2–3% of people taking it) and other neurological adverse effects.

2.4.2.4 Management of chronic liver disease
- Avoid alcohol. Alcohol consumption by an HCV-infected DU/IDU has a significant adverse effect on the course of the liver disease and hence counselling and treatment for alcohol use is strongly indicated.
- Avoid drugs that are toxic to the liver.
- Avoid constipation.

Refer to a specialist if there are complications such as cirrhosis, hepatic encephalopathy and hepatic failure.

> **PRACTICAL POINTS**
> - Treatment of hepatitis C is complex, expensive and requires referral to a specialist.
> - PHCS should monitor the progression of liver disease in IDUs with viral hepatitis by estimating the levels of alanine aminotransferase (ALT) periodically.
> - The primary advice to HBV/HIV or HCV/HIV coinfected individuals should be to avoid alcohol.

2.4.3 Respiratory tract infections

Respiratory tract infections are among the most frequent sequelae of drug use.

■ Risk factors
- DUs have a 10-fold greater risk of community-acquired pneumonia.
- Tobacco smoking is common and hence respiratory clearance mechanisms may be impaired.
- DUs are at an increased risk for aspiration, particularly during overdose.
- An immunocompromised state resulting from HIV infection or poor nutrition may also contribute to the increased risk of respiratory tract infection.
- Inhaling or snorting drugs predisposes DUs to upper respiratory tract infections, including sinusitis and, in rare instances, nasal septum abscesses.

■ Clinical features

Cough and difficulty in breathing are common symptoms in respiratory tract infections (Table 9).

Respiratory rate is a key sign that requires observation:
- 20–30 breaths per minute: fast breathing
- >30 breaths per minute: very fast breathing

Table 9. Signs and symptoms of common respiratory disorders

Signs and symptoms	Possible respiratory problem
Any two of the three: 1. 20–30 breaths per minute 2. Chest pain 3. Night sweats	Pneumonia
Any one or more of the following: • >30 breaths per minute • Temperature 39°C or above • Pulse 120 beats/minute or more • Uncomfortable at rest • Severe chest pain • Lethargy • Unable to walk without assistance	Severe pneumonia
Cough or difficulty in breathing >2 weeks or Recurrent episodes of cough or difficulty in breathing that • wakes the patient in the night, or • in the early morning, or • occurs with exercise	Possible chronic lung problem
Insufficient signs for the above	Consider bronchitis

■ Special features of respiratory tract infections among DUs
- A thorough medical history should be taken (e.g. risk factors for aspiration).
- Atypical clinical findings are common, such as vague chest pain and no fever.
- Atypical radiographic findings are common – consolidation may not be present.
- Aspiration is related to intoxication and overdose.
- Aspiration pneumonia as well as pneumonia caused by *Streptococcus pneumoniae, Haemophilus influenzae, Staphylococcus aureus* and *Klebsiella pneumoniae* are among the most common reasons for admission to a hospital.
- Endovascular infections can cause septic pulmonary emboli that produce pneumonia and lung abscess.

Treatment

Mild-to-moderate community-acquired pneumonia

- *First-line antibiotic*: Common choice: co-trimoxazole. Do not use if the patient is already taking co-trimoxazole preventive therapy as it is likely that the infecting organisms will be resistant to co-trimoxazole.
- *Second-line antibiotic*: Common choice: amoxicillin or macrolides such as erythromycin.

Table 10. Treatment of pneumonia in drug users

Weight	Ampicillin or amoxicillin Give 3 times daily for 5 days		Erythromycin Give 4 times daily for 5 days	
	Tablet 500 mg	Tablet 250 mg	Tablet 500 mg	Tablet 250 mg
<50 kg	1/2	1	1/2	1
>50 kg	1	2	1	2

Severe pneumonia
- *First-line therapy*: cloxacillin + gentamicin IV (*see* section 2.3.1 and Table 5)
- *Second-line therapy*: ceftriaxone IV (*see* section 2.3.1 on treatment of septicaemia) or clindamycin 2400 mg/day in four divided doses at 6-hour intervals
- **PLUS** refer to a hospital.

Aspiration pneumonia
- Treatment is the same as that for severe pneumonia, with the addition of metronidazole 500 mg IV twice daily to the regimen.

Bronchitis
- Amoxicillin (500 mg tablet) 2 tablets twice daily for 7 days or amoxicillin 1 g three times daily IM/IV and change to oral treatment as soon as possible.
- Amoxicillin is the preferred drug but if it is not available it could be replaced with ampicillin.
- If there is no response, then give ampicillin plus gentamicin IV (ampicillin 1 g three times daily + gentamicin 5 mg/kg); change to oral treatment as soon as possible.

Other upper respiratory infections
- Any of the following medications can be used. Note that many upper respiratory tract infections are of viral origin and antibiotics will be ineffective.
  - Amoxicillin (500 mg tablet twice daily for 7 days)
  - Erythromycin (2 g/day in 2–3 divided doses for 7 days) or roxithromycin (150 mg twice daily for 7 days)
  - Azithromycin (500 mg once daily for 3 days)

2.4.4 Tuberculosis (TB)

Globally, it is estimated that about two billion people are infected with *Mycobacterium tuberculosis*, the cause of TB.[23] Most of 9.2 million incident cases of TB occur in developing countries.[24] Tuberculosis is common in both HIV-infected as well as HIV-uninfected DUs. **TB is the most common AIDS-defining illness** and the most common cause of death among people living with HIV (PLHIV) in the developing world.

Pulmonary tuberculosis (PTB) is the commonest form of TB. Lung lesions can be of the following nature: cavities usually in the upper lobes, infiltrates, fibrosis or progressive pulmonary and endobronchial disease. Extrapulmonary tuberculosis (EPTB) is more likely to occur in IDUs, particularly HIV-positive IDUs. The common forms of EPTB associated with HIV include lymphadenopathy, pleural effusion, pericardial disease, miliary TB and meningitis. Many patients with EPTB also have coexistent PTB.

2.4.4.1 Pulmonary tuberculosis (PTB)

■ Risk factors
- Overcrowding and poorly ventilated working and living accommodation
- Among PLHIV there is a 5–10% annual risk of developing TB disease
- Poor nutrition

■ Clinical features

Most patients with PTB feel unwell and are likely to seek medical advice at

some stage. The most important clinical features for the diagnosis of PTB are:
- cough for more than two to three weeks
- sputum production, which may be blood-stained
- weight loss.

Cough is a common symptom, and occurs in over 90% of patients with smear-positive PTB fairly soon after the onset of the disease. Cough is not specific for TB, though if a cough persists for more than three weeks TB should be investigated, particularly in areas where TB is common. Other respiratory symptoms include haemoptysis, chest wall pain and breathlessness.

Generalized, systemic or constitutional symptoms include fever, night sweats, tiredness, loss of appetite and weight loss, which may be substantial. Patients with TB/HIV coinfection have greater weight loss and more prolonged fever than HIV-negative patients. Cough and haemoptysis are symptoms reported less frequently in HIV-positive patients.

The physical signs in patients with PTB are not specific to TB. There may be general signs such as fever, tachycardia (fast pulse rate) and clubbing of the fingers. Chest signs may include crackles, wheezing, and bronchial and amphoric breathing. Usually, there are no abnormal signs in the chest. Consider TB in DUs presenting with pneumonia, and those with known or suspected HIV infection. A purified protein derivative (PPD) test is not useful in this situation as it may be negative if the patient is HIV-positive. Hilar or mediastinal lymphadenopathy on X-ray may be the only finding.

■ Diagnosis

Send three sputum samples for acid-fast bacilli (AFB) if any of the following are present:
- Cough for more than two to three weeks
- Weight loss
- Sputum production.

Screen for TB if a family member has PTB.

Collection of sputum samples

Secretions build up in the airways overnight. Hence, an early morning sputum sample is more likely to contain TB bacilli than one taken later in the day. It may be difficult for an outpatient to provide three early morning sputum samples. Therefore, in practice, an outpatient usually provides sputum samples as follows:

Day 1 sample 1	Patient provides an "on-the-spot" sample under supervision when presenting to the health facility. Give the patient a sputum container to take home for an early morning sample the following morning.
Day 2 sample 2	Patient brings an early morning sample.
Day 2 sample 3	Patient provides another "on-the-spot" sample under supervision.

Some patients cannot produce a sputum sample. A nurse or health worker may need to help them cough and bring up some sputum.

■ Prevention

Isoniazid preventive therapy (IPT)
- IPT seeks to eradicate inactive TB already present in asymptomatic individuals.
- IPT is effective in HIV-positive DUs in settings with low levels of isoniazid (INH) resistance (<10%).
- It is essential to exclude active TB through clinical and laboratory examinations before making a decision to provide IPT.
- Adherence to IPT for those eligible should be ensured through provision of directly observed treatment (DOT).
- IPT can be effectively linked with OST.

- In HIV-infected individuals IPT is more effective with concurrent ART.
- The recommended duration of treatment is 6–9 months at a daily dose of 5 mg per kg body weight (maximum of 300 mg per day).

■ Treatment

WHO recommends the same treatment regimen among TB patients, whether HIV-positive or negative.[25] Treatment regimens have an initial (intensive) phase lasting two months and a continuation phase usually lasting 4–6 months. In the initial phase, usually four drugs are given. In the continuation phase, fewer drugs are necessary but for a longer time. Recommended treatment regimens for TB diagnostic Category 1 patients are two months of, for example, isoniazid (H), rifampicin (R), pyrazinamide (Z) and ethambutol (E), or 2 HRZE in the initial phase, and 4 months of H and R or 6 months of H and E daily in the continuation phase. The latter regimen may be associated with a higher rate of treatment failure and relapse compared with the six-month regimen with rifampicin in the continuation phase. Thiacetazone should not be used for HIV-positive patients. The vast majority of patients with sputum smear-positive TB becomes non-infective within two weeks of treatment (with rifampicin) (Tables 11 and 12).

Table 11. First-line antituberculosis drugs

First-line anti-TB drugs (abbreviation)	Mode of action	Potency	Recommended dose (mg/kg body weight)	
			Daily	Intermittent (3 times a week)
Isoniazid (H)	Bactericidal	High	5	10
Rifampicin (R)	Bactericidal	High	10	10
Pyrazinamide (Z)	Bactericidal	Low	25	35
Streptomycin (S)	Bactericidal	Low	15	15
Ethambutol (E)	Bacteriostatic	Low	15	30

Directly observed treatment, short-course (DOTS)
DOTS is the main strategy for the control of TB, including HIV-associated TB. The key to the success of the DOTS strategy is that it places the responsibility of caring for TB patients on health workers, not on patients.

Table 12. Treatment regimens for TB and their indications

Diagnostic category	Patient type	Regimens	
		Intensive phase[a]	Continuation phase[a]
I	New smear-positive PTB New smear-negative PTB with extensive parenchymal involvement Severe concomitant HIV disease Severe forms of EPTB	2 HREZ[b]	4 HR 6 HE[c]
II	Previously treated sputum smear-positive PTB: • Relapse • Treatment failure[d] • Treatment after interruption	2 HRZES/1 HRZE	5 HRE
III	New smear-negative PTB (other than in Category 1); less severe forms of EPTB	2 HREZ[e]	4 HR 6 HE[c]
IV	Chronic and multidrug-resistant (MDR)-TB cases (still sputum-positive after supervised re-treatment)	Specially designed standardized or individualized regimens are suggested for this category.	

Diagnostic category	Patient type	Regimens	
		Intensive phase[a]	Continuation phase[a]

a. Direct observation of drug intake is required during the initial phase of treatment in smear-positive cases, and always in treatment that includes rifampicin.
b. Streptomycin (provided that sterile syringes and needles, and sharps disposal are available), may be used instead of ethambutol. In meningeal TB, ethambutol should be replaced by streptomycin.
c. This regimen may be associated with a higher rate of treatment failure and relapse compared with the six-month regimen with rifampicin in the continuation phase.
d. Whenever possible, drug sensitivity testing is recommended before prescribing Category II treatment for failure cases. It is recommended that patients with proven MDR-TB use Category IV regimens.
e. Ethambutol may be omitted during the initial phase of treatment for patients with non-cavitary, smear-negative PTB who are known to be HIV-negative, patients known to be infected with fully drug-susceptible bacilli, and young children with primary TB.

Drug interactions between medications for TB, OST and ART

In methadone-maintained DUs, administration of rifampicin produces a significant decrease in methadone levels and induces methadone withdrawal. Hence, an increase in the dose of methadone may be required. Clinical evidence suggests there is little interaction between rifampicin and buprenorphine. Rifampicin reduces NVP levels; the virological consequences of this are uncertain and the potential for additive hepatotoxicity exists. Careful monitoring is required during co-administration.

Rifampicin should not be co-administered with nelfinavir (NFV) and saquinavir (SQV) as it reduces their blood levels.

> **PRACTICAL POINT**
> All PTB patients including those who are HIV-positive should be treated according to the national TB DOTS strategy. This includes the recording and reporting of case detection and treatment outcomes.

2.4.5 HIV

2.4.5.1 HIV testing and counselling

HIV testing and counselling may be client-initiated (CITC) or provider-initiated (PITC). Voluntary and confidential HIV testing and counselling should be routinely offered to all DUs who are at high risk of having HIV infection. While in some situations clients themselves request HIV testing and counselling, health providers are also uniquely placed to routinely offer this service to all those who may be at risk, even when the client has not requested it. PITC can occur in a number of settings such as health facilities, OST programmes, needle and syringe programmes, drug rehabilitation centres and through peer referral.

HIV testing and counselling comprises three steps:
1. Pre-test information and education (group or individual) and provision of individual pre-test counselling if requested
2. Informed consent and HIV testing
3. Post-test counselling.

■ **Pre-test information and education**
- Do a risk assessment for exposure to HIV.
- Assess psychosocial well-being.
- Provide information about HIV/AIDS (including written information) and the implications of testing.

■ **Informed consent and HIV testing**
- Reinforce confidentiality and that testing is voluntary.
- Obtain informed consent.
- Test for HIV (rapid test or enzyme-linked immunosorbent assay [ELISA]).

Additional information with the option of referral should also be available.

■ **Post-test counselling**

If the tests result confirms that the person is *HIV-positive* as per the national

HIV testing strategies, post-test counselling should be offered as follows:
- A confirmed positive result means that the person has HIV infection.
- Break the news sensitively, assessing the capacity to manage the news.
- Provide time for discussion.
- Provide ongoing counselling and care in an arranged follow-up visit.
- Advise about the importance of safe sex, including condom promotion, to prevent transmission of HIV and other STIs.
- Advise about safe injecting practices to prevent transmission of HIV and other bloodborne viruses.
- Develop a risk reduction plan with the patient.
- Discuss voluntary disclosure to partner(s), and HIV testing and counselling for partner(s) and children.
- Refer the patient for HIV prevention, care and treatment services catering to DUs (harm-reduction programmes/drug treatment programmes/opioid substitution programmes/ART programmes), peer support and other appropriate services, as required.
- Refer pregnant patients for prophylaxis to services providing appropriate interventions.

If the result is negative
- Emphasize that a further test is necessary due to the "window period" to ensure an HIV-negative status. The new tests have a narrower window period of two weeks.
- Provide HIV prevention counselling including to partners and reinforce the importance of continued safe sex and safe injecting practices. Promote and provide condoms. If the patient is currently injecting, ensure that they are linked to facilities providing equipment for this. Develop a risk reduction plan with the patient.
- Refer the patient for HIV prevention and care services catering to DUs (harm-reduction programmes/drug treatment programmes/substitution programmes), peer support and other appropriate services, as required.
- Counsel on the need for further HIV testing consistent with the risk assessment profile.

If the result is inconclusive
- Explain what this means.
- Enquire about recent symptoms suggestive of seroconversion illness.
- Provide HIV prevention counselling including to partners and reinforce the importance of continued safe sex and safe injecting practices.
- Re-test in 14 days.
- HIV testing procedures should follow each country's national HIV testing guidelines and algorithms.
- The window period is narrower with the new HIV tests. Risk reduction counselling should be provided to all DUs.
- Refer to the *Guidance on testing and counselling in settings attended by people who inject drugs: improving access to treatment, care and prevention* (WHO, 2008) for further information.[26]

> PRACTICAL POINT = THE THREE Cs
> HIV testing should always
> - Be conducted only with CONSENT, i.e. both informed and voluntary.
> - HIV testing should always be accompanied by COUNSELLING.
> - The HIV test result should be disclosed only to the client ensuring CONFIDENTIALITY of the test result.

Figure 5. HIV testing algorithm

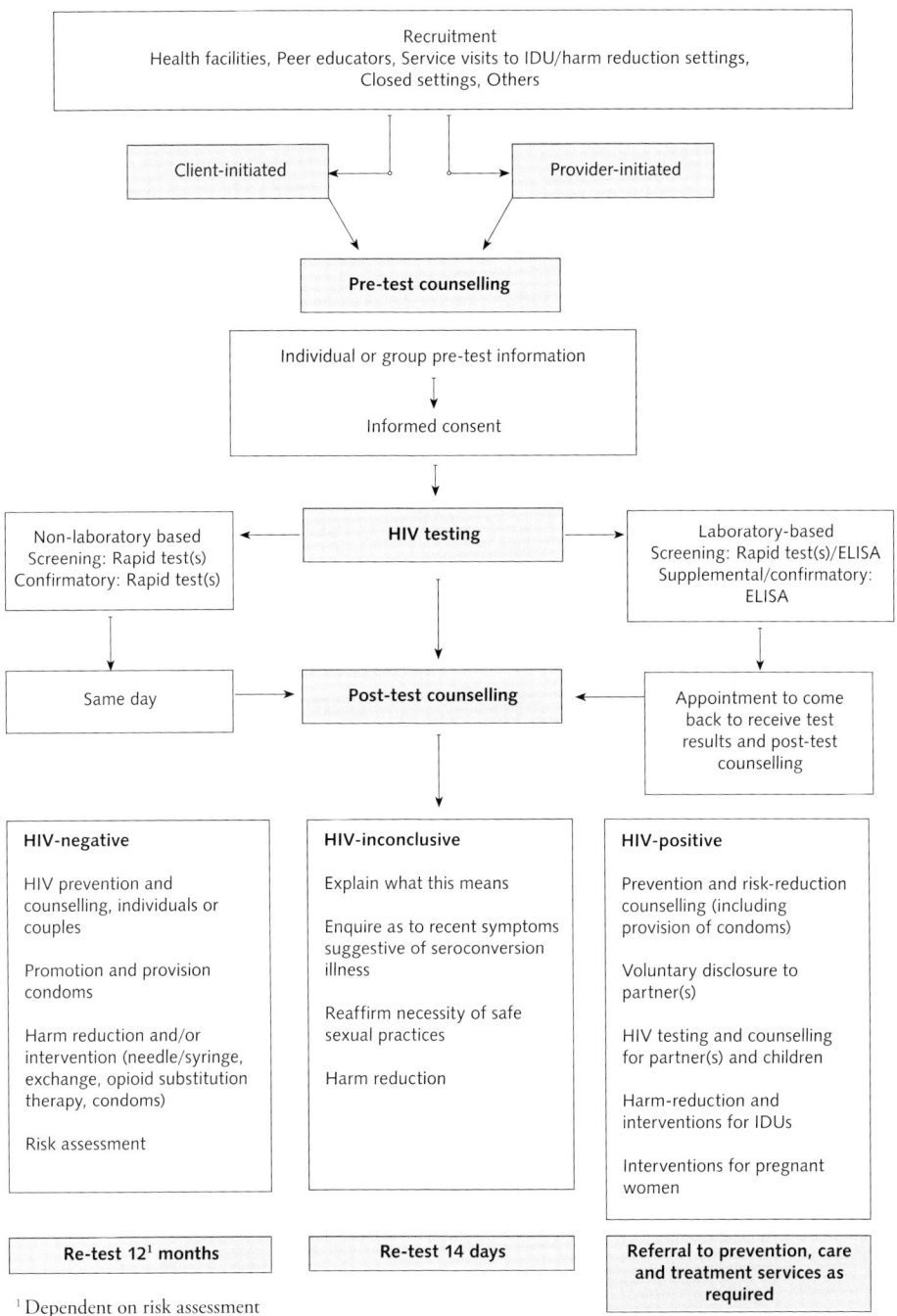

Source: *Guidance on testing and counselling for HIV in settings attended by people who inject drugs: improving access to treatment, care and prevention.* Manila, WHO, 2009.[26]

2.4.5.2 Opportunistic infections

Infections that attack the body only when the immune system is weak are called opportunistic infections (OIs). The hallmark of HIV progression is a decline in CD4 count and eventual increase in viral load. The body is at marked risk for OIs when the CD4 count is <200 cells/mm^3. OIs continue to cause disease and death in patients with HIV infection throughout the world. Rather than HIV itself, it is OIs that cause HIV-related disease and death.

Common OIs include candidiasis, respiratory tract infections such as TB and pneumonia (particularly due to *Pneumocystis jiroveci*), chronic diarrhoea (due to cryptosporidiosis, salmonellosis, amoebiasis, among others), persistent recurrent fever (due to malaria, dengue or HIV-associated infections), malignancies (lymphoma, Kaposi sarcoma), bacterial meningitis, cryptococcal meningitis, toxoplasmosis, among others.

Data from both randomized controlled trials and observational cohort studies have shown that ART is important in preventing the incidence of OIs and improves survival and overall deaths among PLHIV. However, ART does not replace the need for prophylaxis of OIs.[27–31]

■ **Prophylaxis for opportunistic infections**
Co-trimoxazole prophylaxis
Co-trimoxazole prophylaxis may be initiated in two different contexts.[32] "Classic" prophylaxis, where the target is the prevention of *Pneumocystis jiroveci* (earlier known as *carinii*) pneumonia (PCP) and toxoplasmosis, is recommended for all HIV-infected adults with WHO stages 2, 3 and 4 HIV disease or with a CD4 count <200 cells/mm^3 (if available). If the targets of prophylaxis are the reduction in morbidity and mortality associated with bacterial infections and malaria, in addition to the prevention of PCP and toxoplasmosis, co-trimoxazole is recommended for HIV-infected adults with a CD4 count <350 cells/mm^3 or with the same clinical criteria (WHO stage 2, 3 or 4).

Table 13. Summary of recommendations for co-trimoxazole prophylaxis[32]

Key considerations	CD4 count not available	CD4 count available*
When to commence primary co-trimoxazole prophylaxis	WHO clinical stages 2, 3, 4, (including all patients with TB)	Any WHO clinical stage and CD4 <350 cells/mm³ where the aim of co-trimoxazole prophylaxis is the reduction in morbidity and mortality associated with malaria, bacterial diarrhoeal disease and bacterial pneumonias, in addition to the prevention of PCP and toxoplasmosis
Commencing secondary co-trimoxazole prophylaxis	Secondary prophylaxis is recommended for all patients who have completed successful treatment for PCP.	
Timing the initiation of co-trimoxazole in relation to initiating ART	Start co-trimoxazole prophylaxis first. Start ART two weeks later if the individual tolerates co-trimoxazole and has no symptoms of allergy (rash, hepatotoxicity). A two-week gap will assist in clinical management where the cause of the symptoms may be either co-trimoxazole or ART (especially if starting an NVP-containing regimen).	
Universal option	Countries may choose to adopt universal co-trimoxazole prophylaxis for everyone living with HIV and active TB at any CD4 count or clinical stage in settings with a high prevalence of HIV among TB patients and limited health infrastructure.	
Doses of co-trimoxazole in adults and adolescents	One double-strength tablet or two single-strength tablets once daily Total daily dose is 960 mg (800 mg sulfamethoxazole [SMZ] + 160 mg trimethoprim [TMP])	
Co-trimoxazole in pregnant women	Women who fulfil the criteria for co-trimoxazole prophylaxis should continue on it throughout their pregnancy.[33] If a woman requires co-trimoxazole prophylaxis during pregnancy, it should be started regardless of the stage of pregnancy.[34] Breastfeeding women should continue to receive co-trimoxazole prophylaxis.	

Table 13 (*contd*). Summary of recommendations for co-trimoxazole prophylaxis[32]

Key considerations	CD4 count not available	CD4 count available*
Patients allergic to sulfa-based medications	Dapsone 100 mg per day, if available. Co-trimoxazole desensitization may be attempted but not in patients with a previous severe reaction to co-trimoxazole or other sulfa-containing drugs. Refer to *Management of HIV infection and antiretroviral therapy in adults and adolescents* (WHO, 2007) for co-trimoxazole desensitization.[35]	
Monitoring	No specific laboratory monitoring is required in patients receiving co-trimoxazole.	
When to stop prophylaxis (co-trimoxazole or dapsone) in patients on ART	*Option 1* Continue prophylaxis indefinitely *Option 2* Consider discontinuation after one year in patients on ART without WHO stage 2, 3 or 4 events, good adherence and secure access to ART.	CD4 count >200 cells/mm³ for 6 months on ART[36,37]

* Any WHO clinical stage and CD4 count <200 cells/mm³ where the aim of co-trimoxazole prophylaxis is the prevention of *Pneumocystis jiroveci* pneumonia (PCP) and toxoplasmosis, and regular CD4 measurement is possible.

■ Prophylaxis for cryptococcal infection

This should be considered in countries where cryptococcal meningitis is a common OI and fluconazole is available and affordable.

Table 14. Summary of prophylaxis for cryptococcal infection

	When to start	What to start	When to stop
Primary prophylaxis	CD4 count <100 cells/mm³ OR WHO stage 4	Fluconazole 400 mg once weekly	CD4 count >100 cells/mm³ at two consecutive measurements and on ART
Secondary prophylaxis	After successful treatment of cryptococcal infection	Fluconazole 200 mg once daily	If CD4 count measurement not available, do not stop

A syndromic approach to the treatment of OIs is recommended. Commonly encountered symptoms and the likely diagnosis include the following:
- Difficulty in swallowing: oral and oesophageal candidiasis
- Respiratory infections: PTB and PCP are the most common; staphylococcal pneumonia
- Chronic diarrhoea: infectious causes such as amoebiasis, salmonellosis, cryptosporidiosis
- Lymphadenopathy: infections (bacterial or fungal), malignancies
- Persistent recurrent fever: malaria, dengue, skin-related infections, bacteraemia and septicaemia
- Headache and neurological abnormalities: toxoplasmosis, cryptococcal meningitis, bacterial meningitis.

2.4.5.3 Clinical algorithms for the diagnosis and treatment of opportunistic disease

Dysphagia

Figure 6. Management of a patient with difficulty in swallowing

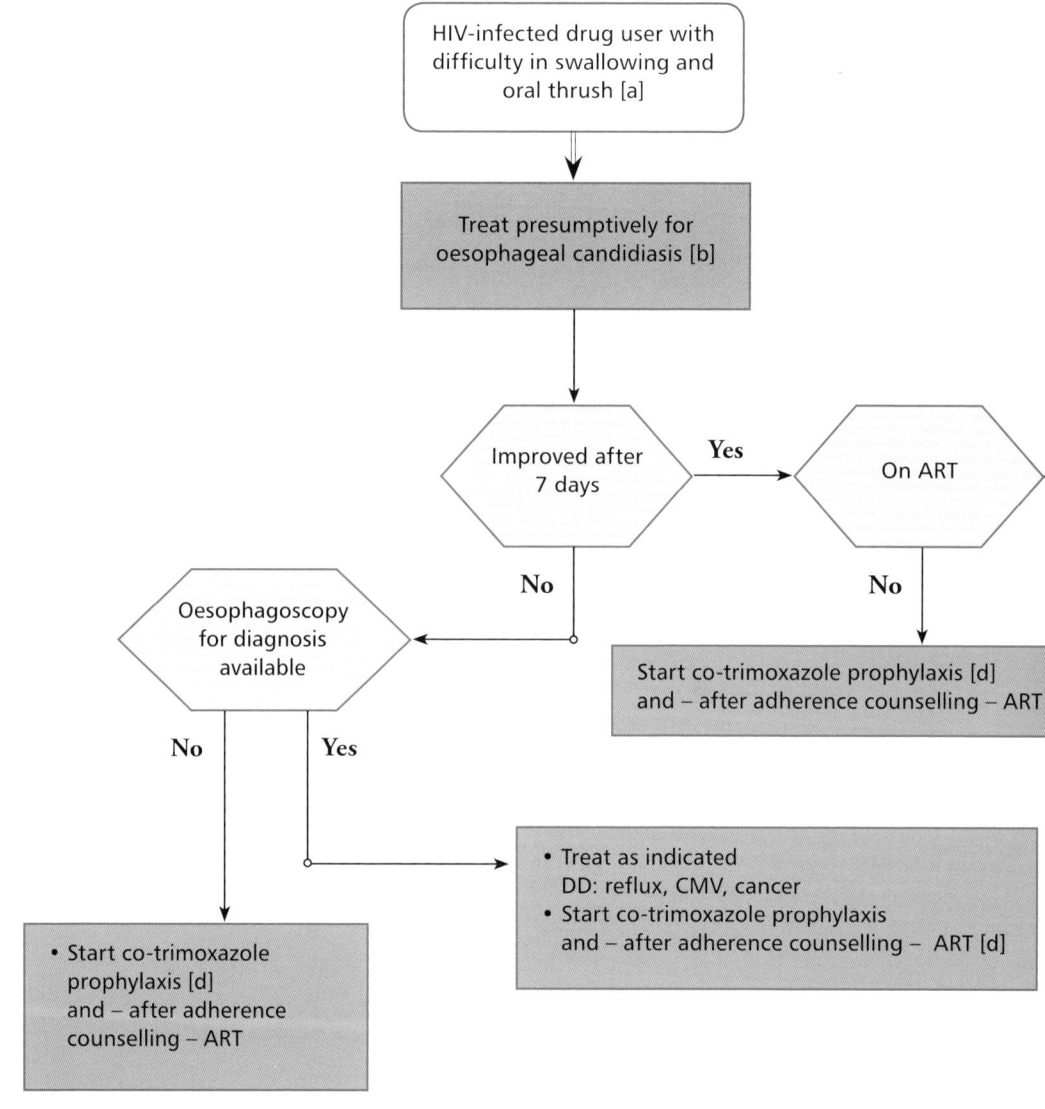

- Continue fluconazole additional 7–14 days
- Check for adherence
- Switch to second-line ART, if failure after ≥6 months first-line therapy
- Start co-trimoxazole prophylaxis
- Consider secondary prophylaxis with fluconazole 200 mg twice weekly [c]

Annotations for Figure 6

a.	**Oral candidiasis** is the most common OI, affecting 75% of patients with HIV infection at some stage during the course of their illness. *Clinical feature* White patches in mouth that can be scraped off *Diagnosis* Clinical diagnosis is usually sufficient. Laboratory diagnosis requires microscopic demonstration of pseudohyphae and/or blastospores of *Candida* spp. from mouth scrapings or biopsy using potassium hydroxide preparations. *Treatment* Fluconazole 100 mg, twice a day for 14 days, clotrimazole oral troche 10 mg, 3–5 times per day for 7–14 days after meals or nystatin suspension 4–6 ml 4 times per day or pastilles 4 times per day after meals or amphotericin lozenges 10 mg 4 times per day after meals. Remove dentures before sucking the lozenges/pastilles/taking oral suspension so that all oral mucosa is exposed to the medication. Oral thrush and other *Candida* infections indicate a high risk for occurrence of OIs. Therefore, primary prophylaxis for PCP is strongly recommended.
b.	**Oesophageal candidiasis.** Many patients presenting with oral candidiasis will also have oesophageal involvement. *Clinical features* Oesophageal candidiasis may cause difficulty in swallowing (dysphagia) and/or pain on swallowing (odynophagia). *Additional information* Severe oral thrush with plaques on the tongue, soft and hard palates extending to the pharynx may indicate oesophageal candidiasis even in the absence of dysphagia. Other common causes of oesophagitis are infections with cytomegalovirus (CMV) or herpes simplex virus (HSV) and aphthous ulceration.

b (contd).	Rarely, these symptoms may be due to malignancy (lymphoma, carcinoma) or ulceration due to contact with oral tablets or acid reflux. Untreated oesophageal lesions may worsen an already poor nutritional status even if they cause only mild discomfort, and may alter eating habits. *Treatment* Fluconazole 200 mg once a day for 14–21 days should be given for oesophageal candidasis. Ketoconazole should be avoided in the presence of active liver disease and concurrent use of rifampicin. Itraconazole 400 mg once daily for 14–21 days may be used as an alternative. In severe cases intravenous amphotericin may be given, but this is expensive and may cause acute renal failure. Refractory cases require referral to a specialist.
c.	Oral thrush and oesophageal candidiasis may frequently relapse in the absence of immune reconstitution and prophylaxis after therapy. Regular follow up for symptoms and inspection of the oral cavity are recommended.
d.	Oesophageal candidiasis is considered as WHO clinical stage 4. Therefore, starting co-trimoxazole and ART is indicated.

Respiratory infections

Figure 7. Management of a patient with respiratory infection

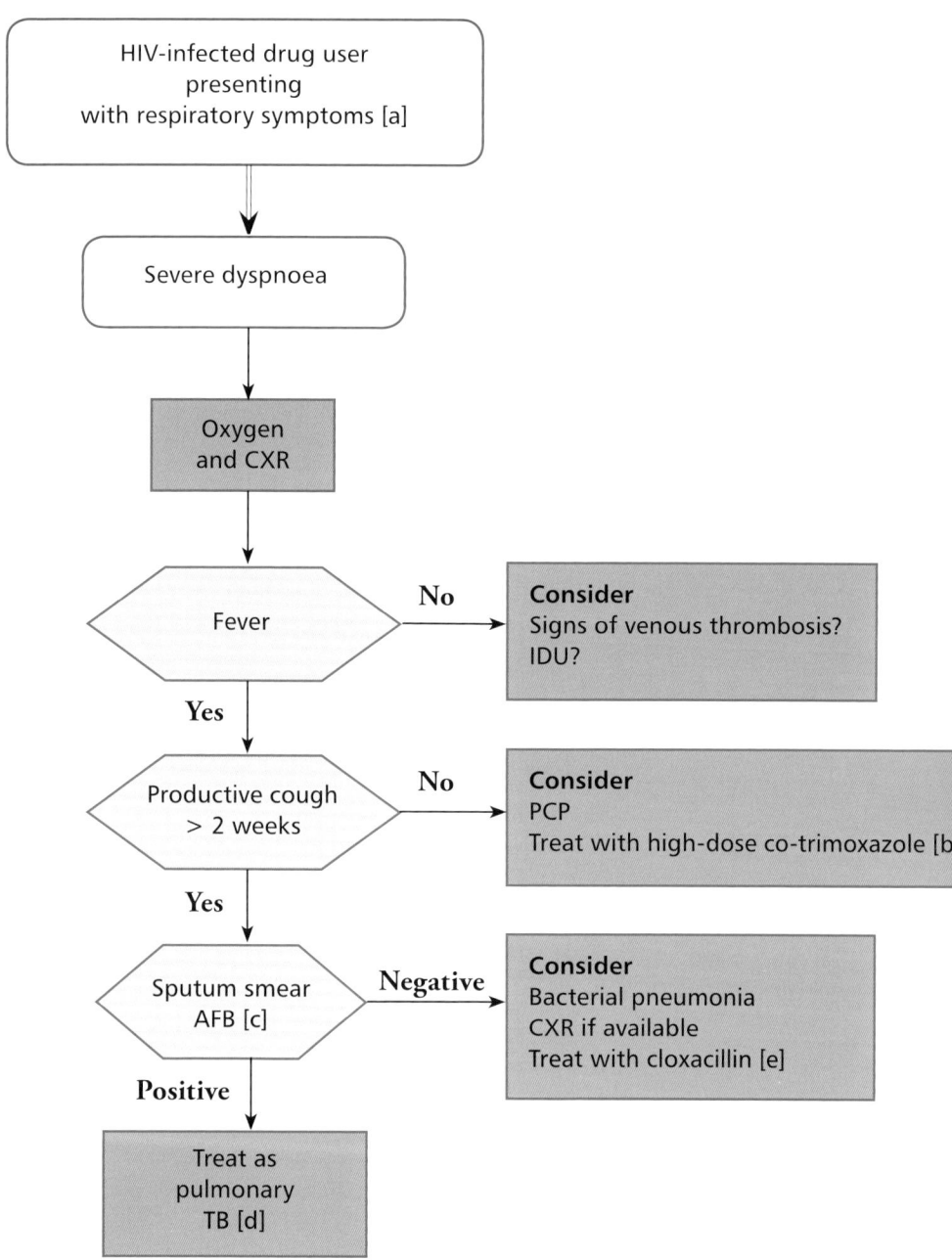

Annotations for Figure 7

a.	Pulmonary tuberculosis (PTB) and *Pneumocystis jiroveci* pneumonia (PCP) are the most common OIs among HIV-infected persons with immunosuppression. Both bacterial pneumonia and PTB are more common in IDUs than non-injecting DUs. Look for • Oxygen level? • Heart murmur? • Clubbing? • Cardiac decompensation? • Auscultation? • Chest X-ray (CXR), if available
b.	The administration of co-trimoxazole prophylaxis for PCP is recommended when the CD4 count is <350 cells/mm^3 or total lymphocyte count (TLC) is <1200 cells. An HIV-infected individual presenting with severe respiratory distress, dry cough and fever, and not currently taking co-trimoxazole will most likely have PCP. After stabilization with oxygen, a CXR should be done immediately. The CXR may be normal in patients with PCP or PTB. Co-trimoxazole (trimethoprim–sulfamethoxazole [TMP–SMZ], dosage calculated as TMP 20–25 mg/kg/day), can be given orally or intravenously in 3–4 divided doses. If the patient is unable to tolerate co-trimoxazole (e.g. due to drug rash), the alternatives are: Clindamycin 300–450 mg orally every 6 hours Pentamidine isetionate 3–4 mg/kg once daily IV Dapsone 100 mg orally once daily + TMP 15 mg/kg/day orally. Prednisolone is recommended in severely ill patients. The regimen used is 40 mg twice a day for 5 days, followed by 20 mg twice a day for 5 days and 20 mg once daily for another 11 days. Assessment of benefit requires at least 4 days. If the patient responds, treatment is continued for at least 21 days. **Prophylaxis for TB should be initiated if prednisolone is used. Supplemental O$_2$ therapy at 6–8 litres/min is advisable.**

Annotations for Figure 7 (contd)

b. (contd)	The risk of recurrence of PCP is high; therefore, secondary prophylaxis with TMP–SMZ single-strength tablet (480 mg) once daily is recommended. Alternative regimens are TMP–SMZ double-strength tablet (960 mg) once daily or dapsone 100 mg once daily.
c.	Sputum examination is important for identifying the etiological agent. The sputum smear should be Gram-stained, inspected for AFB (at least 2 sputum samples should be obtained) and cultured. If the chest X-ray shows a pleural effusion, a pleural aspiration for culture and a pleural biopsy should be performed.
d.	*See* section 2.4.4 for the diagnosis and management of TB.
e.	Staphylococcal pneumonia is a very common form of pneumonia in IDUs, as a result of injection-site infections. Administration of cloxacillin plus gentamicin is therefore recommended (*see* Annex 3).

Chronic diarrhoea

Figure 8. Management of a patient with chronic diarrhoea

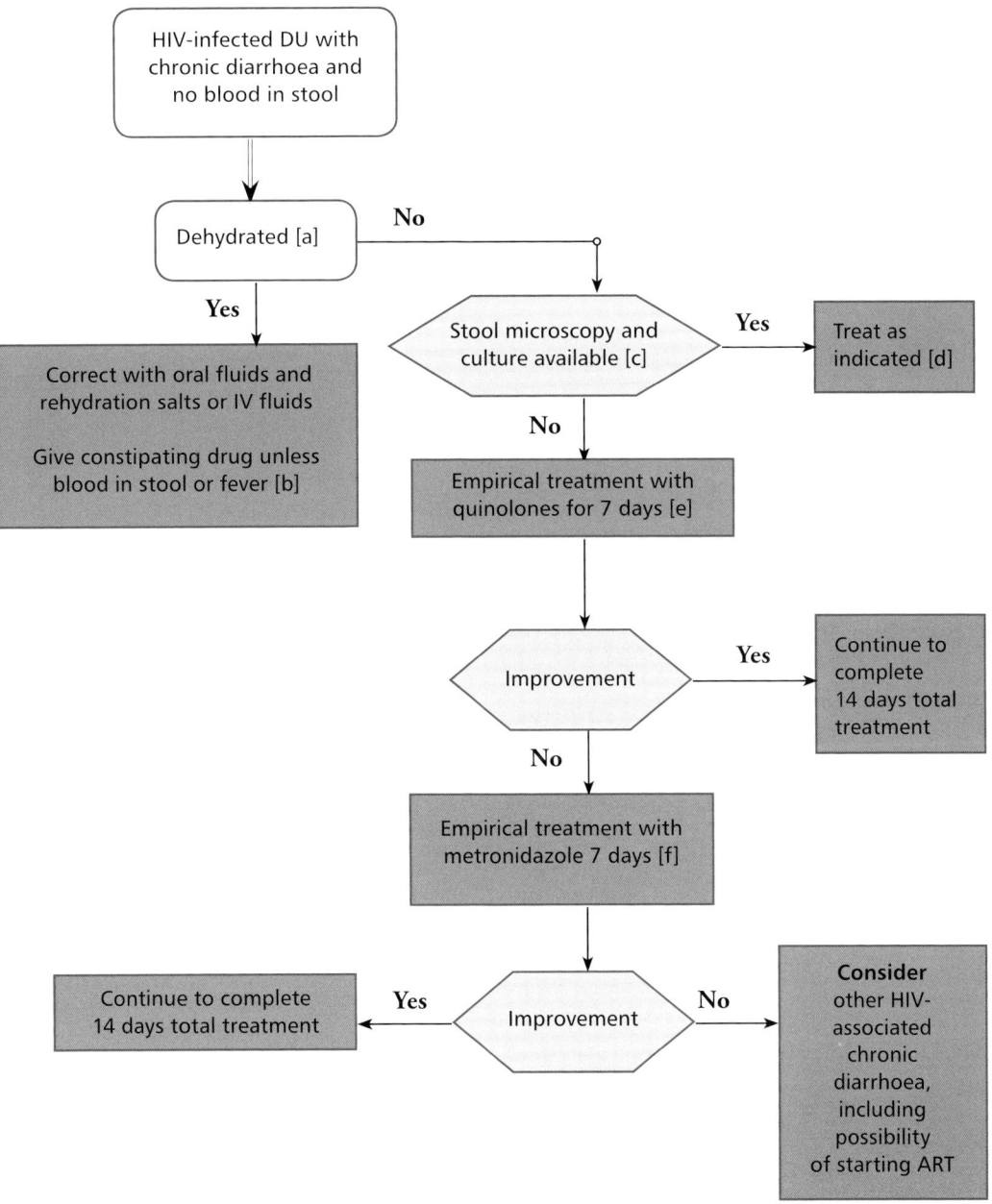

Annotations for Figure 8

a.	All patients with chronic diarrhoea should be encouraged to replace lost fluids using oral rehydration solution (ORS). This can be purchased over the counter at pharmacies or made at home. Frequent intake of small amounts of fluid is recommended.
b.	Treatment of diarrhoea involves either treating the symptoms or the cause. *Treatment of symptoms* Fluids (including ORS) and antimotility agents (e.g. loperamide) *Treatment of the cause* Antibiotics for infectious diarrhoea TB treatment of refractory diarrhoea related to TB infection in the gut Always consider starting ART, particularly in the context of wasting.
c.	The presence of blood, pus or mucus indicates that the diarrhoea is infectious and antibiotics will be needed. Refer to the *Management of HIV infection and antiretroviral therapy in adults and adolescents: a clinical manual* (WHO, 2007) for details of treatment.[35]
d.	If no pathogen is found or the diarrhoea is refractory to treatment, then TB should be considered, particularly if fever is present.
e.	If repeated examinations fail to identify a pathogen, a course of empirical antibiotics should be tried before giving antimotility drugs. Antimotility agents should not be used in patients with bloody diarrhoea because of the risk of inducing toxic megacolon. Typical antimotility agents include loperamide or diphenoxylate. For example, loperamide 4 mg may be given initially, followed by a further 2 mg after 4–12 hours (maximum daily dosage 16 mg/day) or diphenoxylate 5 mg 4 times daily (depending on how well the symptoms are controlled).
f.	Alcohol should be avoided during treatment with metronidazole, because of the risk of a disulfiram-type reaction.

Lymphadenopathy

Figure 9. Management a patient with lymphadenopathy

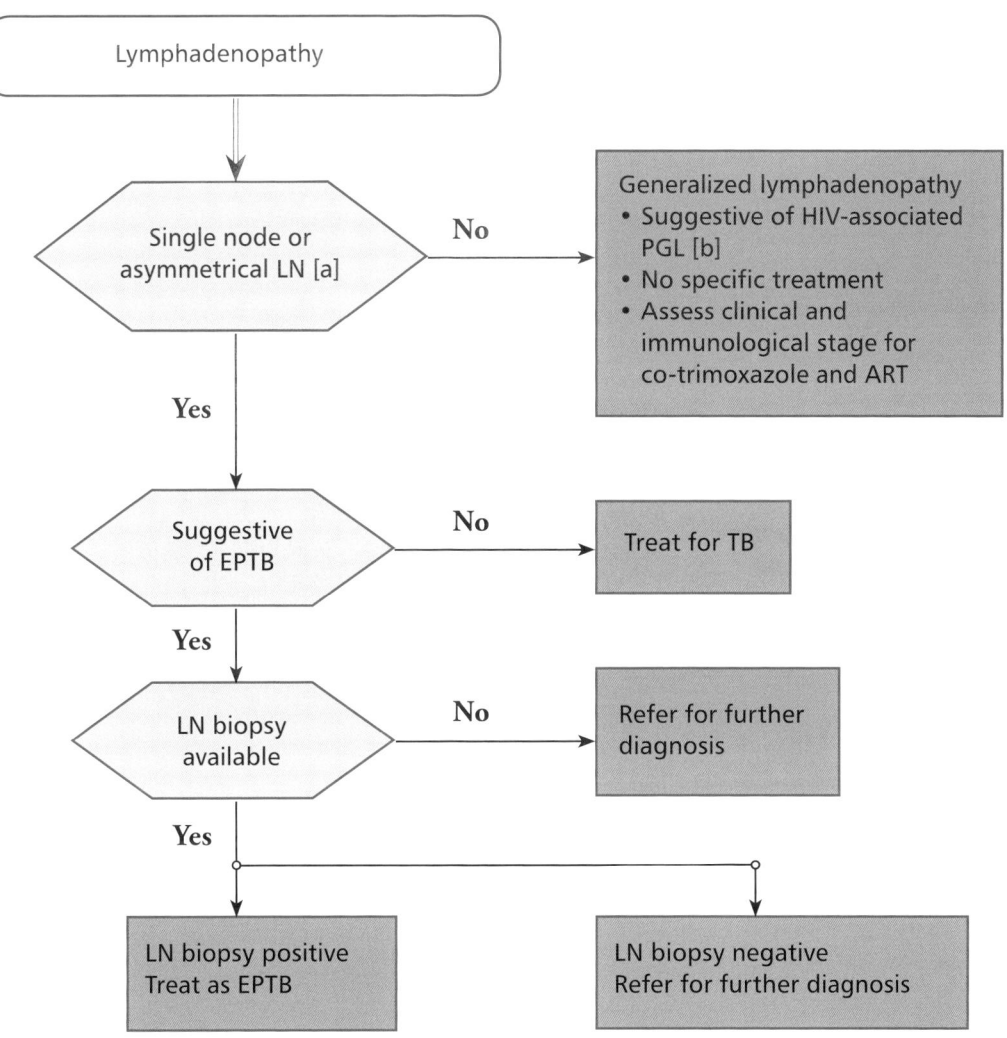

Annotations for Figure 9

a.	Lymph node enlargement in a patient with symptomatic HIV infection can be related to HIV infection alone or more commonly may be caused by other infections or sometimes malignancy.
	• Infections
	  —Bacterial (TB)
	  —Fungal (e.g. cryptococcosis)
	• Malignancies (e.g. lymphoma)
	
	In asymptomatic patients no further investigation or treatment is required. However, in patients with recently symptomatic lymphadenopathy, rapidly enlarging lymph nodes, marked nodal asymmetry and constitutional symptoms, referral for biopsy should be considered. Biopsy is also advised for patients not responding to empirical treatment. Refer to *Management of HIV infection and antiretroviral therapy in adults and adolescents* (WHO, 2007) for further information.[35]

b.	Persistent generalized lymphadenopathy (PGL) is common in asymptomatic HIV-infected patients and is often due to HIV infection alone. It is defined as the following: More than 3 separate lymph node groups affected At least 2 nodes more than 1.0 cm in diameter at each site Duration >1 month No local or contiguous infection that might explain the adenopathy.

Persistent recurrent fever

Figure 10. Management of a patient with persistent recurrent fever

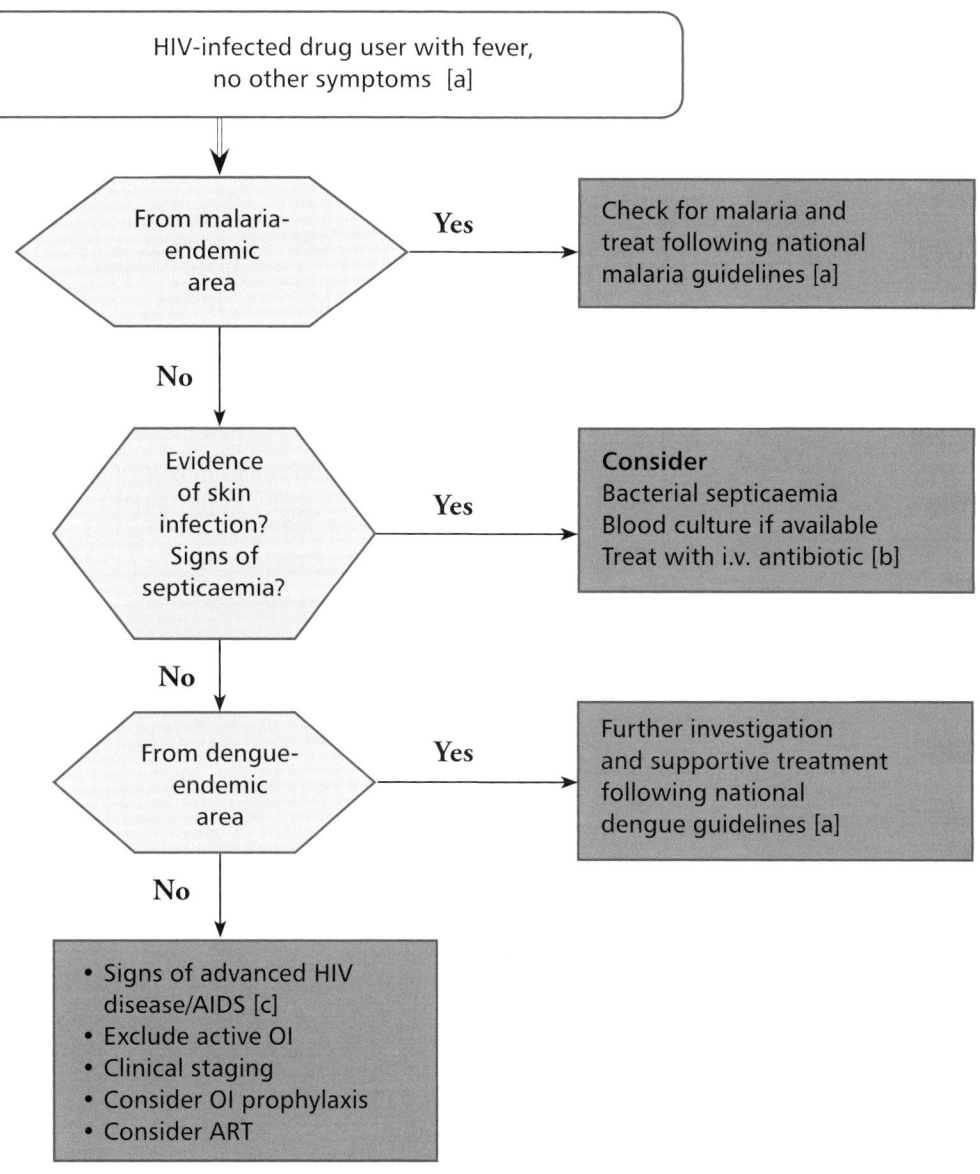

Annotations for Figure 10

a.	Screen for malaria, dengue, skin-related infections and HIV-associated infections.
	Definition
	Fever is defined as a body temperature of ≥37.5°C. Prolonged fever is defined as fever for more than 14 days. A blood smear for malarial parasites should be carried out in areas where the disease is endemic or when there is a history of recent travel to such areas. Treatment regimens for malaria should follow national and international recommendations.
b.	When there is evidence of skin-associated infection assume bacteraemia or other systemic bacterial complication and treat with broad-spectrum antibiotics such as cloxacillin or amoxicillin with clavulanate for 5/7 days. If there is no response refer for further investigations to rule out other infections.
c.	A full blood count and CD4 count should be carried out as part of the assessment. Isolation of bacteria from various specimens as clinically indicated is recommended. *Salmonella* bacteraemia is more common in HIV-infected patients. Screen for mycobacterial infection. For further information refer to *Management of HIV infection and antiretroviral therapy in adults and adolescents: a clinical manual* (WHO, 2007).[35]

Common health problems associated with drug use/injecting drug use

Headache and neurological abnormalities

Figure 11. Management of a patient with headache and neurological abnormalities

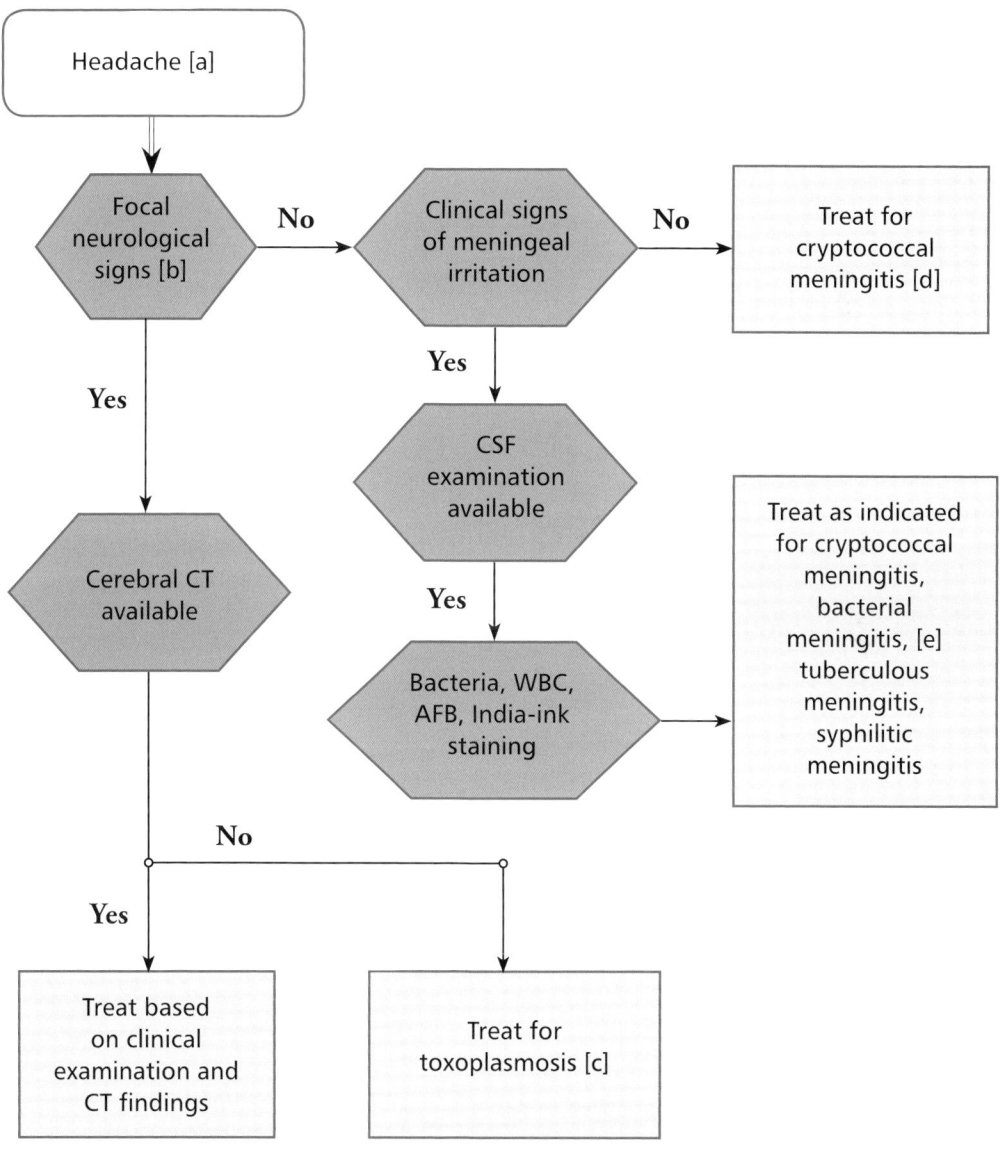

Management of common health problems of drug users

Annotations for Figure 11

a.	Causes of headache include cryptococcal meningitis, tuberculous meningitis, cerebral toxoplasmosis, chronic HIV meningitis, bacterial meningitis and lymphoma. Causes of headache not related to HIV infection include migraine, syphilis, tension, sinusitis, refractive disorders, dental disease, anaemia and hypertension. Other infectious diseases such as malaria, typhoid fever, dengue fever and rickettsiosis can also cause headache.
b.	Neurological examination • Evidence of meningeal irritation (photophobia, neck stiffness) or raised intracranial pressure (high blood pressure and slow pulse in the presence of fever) • Changes in mental state • Focal neurological deficits including paresis, cranial nerve palsies, movement disorders, ataxia, aphasia and seizures
c.	*Toxoplasmosis* Pyrimethamine loading dose 75–100 mg, then 25–50 mg daily plus sulfadiazine 4 g daily in 4 divided doses for 6 weeks followed by chronic suppressive therapy with pyrimethamine, 25 mg daily plus sulfadiazine 2 g daily in 4 divided doses. Alternative therapy is pyrimethamine as above plus clindamycin 300 mg four times a day for 6 weeks.
d.	*Cryptococcal meningitis*
e.	*Bacterial meningitis* Benzyl penicillin 1.2–2.4 million IU daily by IV injection in divided doses every 4 hours. Treat for a minimum of 7 days or for 4–5 days after the patient becomes afebrile. If the patient is allergic to penicillin, ampicillin or chloramphenicol or ceftriaxone can be used.

For row d, the cryptococcal meningitis treatment table:

Primary treatment	*Maintenance treatment*
Amphotericin B 0.7–1 mg/kg/day IV for 14 days + itraconazole 200 mg 2 times daily for 8 weeks or fluconazole 400 mg daily for 8–12 weeks	Amphotericin B 0.7–1 mg/kg/week
	Itraconazole 200 mg/day or fluconazole 200 mg/day

2.4.5.4 Immune reconstitution inflammatory syndrome (IRIS)

IRIS is a collection of symptoms and signs as a result of immune recovery on ART.[38] It can present as a paradoxical worsening of clinical disease after initial improvement following several weeks of therapy, with the signs and symptoms of a previously subclinical and unrecognized OI or as an autoimmune disease. Typically, IRIS occurs within 2–12 weeks of initiation of ART, although it may present later.

IRIS has been reported in association with a large number of HIV-related infections and inflammatory conditions, the most frequent being mycobacterial disease (TB or *Mycobacterium avium* complex [MAC]) and cryptococcal disease. Together, these account for about 60% of all cases of IRIS in developed country settings.[39]

Hepatic flares may occur during ART in HBV/HIV coinfection as a presentation of IRIS. They are characterized by an acute rise in hepatic transaminases accompanied by symptoms of acute hepatitis (fatigue, abdominal pain and jaundice). These reactions generally occur in the first few months of treatment and may be difficult to distinguish from ART-induced hepatotoxicity. In such cases, all ARV drugs should be withheld until the clinical condition improves.

■ Risk factors
- Initiating ART in the presence of signs and symptoms of an OI
- Being ART-naive at the time of presentation of an OI
- Initiating ART when the CD4 count is <50 cells/mm^3
- Having a more rapid initial decrease in the HIV-1 RNA level in response to ART than in patients with higher CD4 counts.

■ Clinical features
- May be mild and resolve without treatment (e.g. mild rash and fever or a transient rise in hepatic enzymes)

- May be severe and life-threatening, as in patients with cryptococcal meningitis or TB

■ Management of IRIS
- Rule out new OIs.
- Rule out drug toxicity.
- If IRIS is suspected, is it a
  - manifestation of a new or ongoing infection (early presentation)?
  - reconstitution immune reaction to non-replicating antigens (late presentation)?
- Avoid interruption of ART.
- Treat with antimicrobials if new infection is suspected and continue previous therapy.
- Treat with anti-inflammatory medications such as NSAIDs and corticosteroids (no definitive protocol though clinicians use prednisone 1 mg/kg/day with tapering over several weeks).

Table 15. Immune reconstitution inflammatory syndrome

Definition	A collection of signs and symptoms resulting from the ability to mount an immune response associated with immune recovery on ART[38]
Frequency	10% of all patients initiating ART In patients initiating ART with a CD4 cell count <50 cells/mm^3 the frequency is up to 25%.[40,41]
Timing	Typically within 2–12 weeks of initiation of ART but may present later
Signs and symptoms	The most common IRIS events are infection with *M. tuberculosis*, *Mycobacterium avium* complex (MAC) or cryptococcal disease[39] and hepatitis B. Unexpected deterioration of clinical status soon after commencing ART Unmasking of subclinical infections, which present as new active disease and/or worsening of coexisting infections
Management	IRIS may be mild and resolve without treatment. Continue ART if the patient can tolerate it. Treat unmasked active OIs such as TB.

For further details, refer to *Treatment and care for HIV-positive drug users: module 6.5* (ASEAN/USAID/WHO/FHI, 2007).[42]

2.5 Non-infectious disorders

2.5.1 Psychiatric disorders

Psychiatric comorbidity and other psychological problems are very common among DUs regardless of the HIV status.

2.5.1.1 Psychiatric disorders in drug users (independent of HIV status)

Common psychiatric disorders
- Major depression
- Bipolar disorder
- Anxiety disorders
- Schizophrenia
- Personality disorders

Substance use-related disorders
- Withdrawal syndromes
- Substance use-related mood disorders (e.g. depression)
- Substance-induced psychosis

The most prevalent psychiatric disorders in those who use substances are depressive disorders.

2.5.1.2 HIV-related psychiatric disorders

Psychological impact of HIV
Primary care providers should be aware of the specific and general factors that may trigger or exacerbate psychological distress or psychiatric disorders in HIV-infected persons and their families.

Crisis points in HIV-infected DUs
- Ongoing psychosocial difficulties associated with drug use
- Learning of HIV-positive status

- Disclosure of HIV or drug-using status to family and friends
- Introduction of ART
- Periods of drug abstinence and withdrawal
- Occurrence of any physical illness
- Recognition of new symptoms/progression of disease, e.g. major drop in CD4 counts, rise in viral load
- Necessity for hospitalization (particularly the first hospitalization)
- Death of a significant other
- Diagnosis of AIDS
- Changes in major aspects of lifestyle, e.g. loss of job, end of relationship, relocation
- Necessity of making end-of-life decisions.

Exacerbation of pre-existing psychiatric disorders can interfere with the ability to cope with HIV infection. HIV is a risk factor for developing a range of psychiatric disorders including
- mood disorders – depression, mania
- anxiety disorders – panic and generalized anxiety disorders
- adjustment disorders
- psychosis
- substance use
- organic mental disorders – cognitive disorders
- HIV-associated delirium and dementia.

Conditions that require referral to specialist services
- Major depression refractory to treatment
- Bipolar disorder
- Schizophrenia
- Suicidal or homicidal thoughts
- Severe cognitive impairment

2.5.1.3 Management of common mental health conditions

Perform an initial comprehensive assessment followed by an annual mental health assessment for all HIV-infected patients.

Depression

Depression is the most common psychiatric comorbidity associated with drug use.

- **Risk factors**
- History of prior mood disorder
- History of anxiety disorder
- Prior suicide attempt
- Family history of depression or suicide
- Inadequate social support
- Non-disclosure of HIV status
- Recent loss (occupation, family)
- Multiple losses
- Advancing illness
- Treatment failure
- Hepatitis C treatment with interferon (IFN)

- **Clinical features**
- Depressed mood
- Lack of interest in pleasurable activities and social withdrawal
- Psychological symptoms
    – crying spells
    – low self-esteem
    – pessimism
    – helplessness
    – hopelessness
    – worthlessness
    – suicidal ideas and/or intent
- Physical symptoms
    – non-specific and generalized aches and pains
    – sleep disturbances
    – reduced energy levels
    – reduced motor activity

- loss of appetite
- constipation
- loss of libido

Depression is often underdiagnosed and undertreated. A family history of depression is common among persons presenting with major depression. Depression can be both a cause and a consequence of substance use.

Depression is common during treatment with interferon for hepatitis C, though this usually resolves after treatment is completed.

It is important for providers to consider alternative diagnostic possibilities for depressive symptoms (e.g. acute medical illness, dementia, substance use-related conditions).

Differentiating appropriate sadness and adjustment issues from pathological depression may be difficult in an HIV-infected person.
- The psychomotor retardation and apathy of AIDS dementia complex may be confused with depression (improves with combination ART).
- Organic mood disorders may also have symptoms similar to major depression (responsive to antidepressant medication).

Patients with depressive symptoms may be at increased risk for transmission of HIV infection due to an increased likelihood of engaging in high-risk behaviours. HIV-infected DUs with depression are less likely to adhere to ART or other treatments (e.g. TB treatment). Treatment of depression increases adherence.

■ Diagnosis
The following questions should be asked by a clinician to assess depression in PHCS.

During the past month:
- Do you feel little interest or pleasure in doing things?

- Have you felt low, depressed, or had thoughts of hopelessness or worthlessness?

Assessment for suicidal risk is crucial when dealing with a patient with depressive symptoms:
- Assess and document suicidal thoughts and intentions
  – Have you ever thought of harming yourself?
  – Have you had these thoughts recently?
  – Have you made a plan to end your life?
  – Do you think you would ever act on these thoughts?
- Closely monitor patients who give answers indicating that they have an intention to harm themselves and refer to psychiatric services.

■ Treatment

Effective management of depression should include co-management of the substance use disorder.
- Pharmacotherapy (medication) is the mainstay of treatment for major depression.
- Drugs used to treat depression are not dependence-inducing (not addictive).
- Drugs take some time to produce a clinical response (up to 3 weeks), but symptoms such as sleep disorder improve within 2–3 days.
- Side-effects usually diminish in 7–10 days.
- Drugs need to be continued for a minimum of six months. The doctor should be consulted before stopping the drugs.
- No single antidepressant is superior in treating HIV-infected patients as a group.
- Patient adherence to regimens is critical.
- Those who take adequate doses of antidepressants have the best chance of improving.
- A general rule is to start with low doses of any medication, titrating up to a full dose slowly, in order to minimize early side-effects that may act as obstacles to adherence.
- Refer cases with severe depression to a psychiatrist.

Table 16. Treatment of depression

Medication	Initial dose	Minimal time between dose increases	Maximum dose increase each time	Maximum	Side-effects
Fluoxetine	10–20 mg daily	2–3 weeks	10 mg	60 mg	Nausea, dyspepsia, headache, insomnia
Amitriptyline	25–75 mg daily 25 mg in the elderly or HIV stage 3 or 4	1 week	25 mg	150–200 mg	Sedation and increased risk of overdose, dry mouth, constipation, urinary retention

Other drugs used for the treatment of depression

Selective serotonin reuptake inhibitors (SSRIs) such as fluoxetine are first-line drugs for the treatment of depression. Other SSRIs are given below.

Citalopram: dose range 20 mg once daily; increase by 10 mg every 2–3 weeks (maximum 60 mg daily)

Sertraline: dose range 50 mg once daily; increase by 50 mg after 2–4 weeks to a maximum of 200 mg daily and then reduce to lowest effective dose.

Mirtazipine: starting dose 15 mg at night and increase to 30–45 mg as tolerated.

The other tricyclic antidepressants that can be used to treat depression include doxepin (10–300 mg/day, dothiepin (75–225 mg/day) and imipramine (25–200 mg/day).

Patients often require substantial education about the disease, nature of their depression, encouragement and therapeutic optimism that the treatment will work. Reducing the stigma associated with depression and its treatment is important in the treatment process. This includes working with family members. In addition to pharmacotherapy, cognitive–behavioural therapy (CBT) may be helpful for depressed individuals.

Anxiety

Anxiety is very commonly associated with substance-use disorders, particularly during withdrawal from opiates and intoxication with amphetamines and other stimulants. It can also occur as an independent condition.

■ Clinical features
- Excessive anxiety and worry
- Psychological symptoms
  - feeling nervous
  - fear for no reason, excessive fear in familiar situations
  - inability to relax
- Physical symptoms
  - restlessness
  - getting easily fatigued
  - difficulty in concentrating or mind going blank
  - irritability
  - tense muscles
  - sleep disturbance

Often, anxiety presents in episodic attacks (panic attacks). Common symptoms in this case are palpitations, tremors, excessive sweating, frequent urination, dry mouth, difficulty in breathing and feeling dizzy.

■ Treatment
- Relaxation techniques (e.g. Jacobson muscle relaxation technique)
- Supportive psychotherapy (reassurance, explanation, expert advice, suggestions, guidance, ventilation, support and facilitating emotional support from key persons)
- Short-term treatment can be given with longer-acting anti-anxiety drugs such as clonazepam 0.25 mg twice daily orally along with psychological therapies. Clonazepam is preferred to shorter-acting benzodiazepines such as lorazepam and alprazolam which are not recommended because of the potential for abuse and dependence. The dose of clonazepam can be increased every three days in increments of 0.125–0.25 mg twice daily.

The target dose for panic disorder is 1.0 mg per day although some people benefit from doses up to a maximum of 4 mg per day. When a person stops taking clonazepam, the drug should be gradually discontinued by decreasing the dose by 0.125 mg twice daily every three days. To prevent any misuse, the prescription should be limited to only the short term; clients on prescription need to be counselled accordingly.
- Drugs such as imipramine (dose: 25–100 mg) or selective serotonin reuptake inhibitors (SSRIs) such as fluoxetine (dose: 10–20 mg) may be useful as medium to long-term therapy, particularly in panic attacks and problematic anxiety disorders.
- For severe cases, refer to a specialist.

Insomnia
- Insomnia is the inability to fall asleep or waking up excessively early.
- It is either primary (no cause) or secondary to other causes (depression, anxiety, psychosis) and is extremely common in DUs.
- Effective treatment involves treating the cause of the insomnia, which may involve addressing the issue of substance use.

■ Treatment
Teach sleep hygiene approaches:
- Increase daily exercise to at least 30 minutes at moderate intensity (not in the evening).
- Avoid daytime napping.
- Avoid caffeine, particularly in the afternoon.
- Reduce alcohol intake.
- Use the bed only for sleeping and sexual activity.
- Use relaxation techniques prior to sleep (e.g. progressive muscle relaxation).
- Develop a regular routine of rising and retiring at the same time each day.

If hypnotics are advised, prescribe them only for a short time.
Efavirenz may cause sleep disturbance in the first few weeks of treatment, though this usually resolves.

Cognitive disturbances

Cognitive disorders include memory disturbances and confusion. Primary care providers should assess for cognitive disturbance.

■ Diagnosis

Items from a standard mini mental exam are useful in screening for cognitive disturbances including delirium (fluctuating level of cognitive impairment) and dementia (permanent memory loss).
- Orientation (name, date and place of examination)
- Registration and recall (three words)
- Language (naming objects)
- General information that may provide additional insight, such as naming the prime minister of the country or four cities in the country.

An organic contribution to aberrant cognition should be considered:
- Substance use-related: intoxication, withdrawal, delirium
- HIV-related central nervous system disorders: toxoplasmosis
- HIV-related cognitive impairment: direct result of HIV infection of the brain
- Psychiatric disorders: depression, psychosis
- Others: infection, hepatic encephalopathy, electrolyte imbalance, hypoxia, subdural haematoma from head trauma.

■ Clinical features

Delirium is characterized by a fluctuating level of consciousness and
- Recent onset of confusion
- Difficulty in speaking
- Disorientation in place or time
- Restlessness and agitation
- Reduced level of consciousness.

In *dementia* the level of consciousness is not reduced but there are other problems such as
- Serious memory problems, or
- Slowed thinking with trouble paying attention, or

- Misplacing important objects, or
- Loss of orientation

Dementia is a chronic, usually progressive problem that does not resolve.

■ Treatment
Delirium
- Consider substance use (alcohol)-related delirium and manage accordingly.
- If the person is agitated and not alcohol- or drug-intoxicated, give low-dose sedation with haloperidol.
- Consider HIV-related illness (if HIV-related, condition improves with ART).

Dementia
- Rule out treatable (reversible) dementias (e.g. hypothyroidism, chronic subdural haematoma, normal-pressure hydrocephalus).
- Rule out pseudodementia (major depression mimics dementia).
- Consider HIV-related illness (if HIV-related, it improves with ART).
- Work closely with family members to advise them of the treatment options and prognosis.

Psychotic disorders

Psychosis is characterized by delusions (false beliefs in the face of evidence against) and hallucinations (the experience of sights and sounds such as voices that are not actually present).

Drug-induced psychosis is commonly associated with amphetamine intoxication, particularly in chronic amphetamine users.

■ Clinical features
- Bizarre and uncooperative behaviour
- Irrelevant, often nonsensical speech
- Agitation and violence
- Auditory hallucinations or internal dialogue

- **Treatment**
- Refer to psychiatric services.
- Emergency management of agitation or violence:
  - Administer haloperidol
    - If medically healthy, give haloperidol IM 5 mg once or twice daily
    - If medically ill, elderly, in HIV clinical stage 3 or 4 then give haloperidol IM 0.5–1 mg once or twice daily
    - In uncontrollable HIV clinical stage 3 or 4 patient: haloperidol 2 mg and, if no response in one hour, repeat haloperidol 2 mg. If still not adequately sedated, add diazepam 2–5 mg orally.
    - Haloperidol can be continued as an oral dose (same dose) if the patient is cooperative.
- Side-effects of haloperidol are stiffness, tremor, muscle spasm, akinesia and motor restlessness. If there is acute muscle spasm, stop haloperidol, maintain airway, give diazepam 5 mg rectally and refer.
- The management of chronic psychosis in IDUs is complex and requires experienced psychiatric care.

2.5.2 Management of harmful and dependent substance use

Substance dependence is a chronic, relapsing medical condition. Dependent users of harmful substances often have many problems related to family, work, social functioning and the law. Illicit drug use is often associated with criminal involvement and subsequent incarceration.

Further, other medical and psychiatric comorbidities are very commonly associated with psychoactive substance use.

As the PHCS will probably be providing services for individuals experiencing complications from heroin, opium or ATS use, an understanding of how these substances can affect the physical and mental health of users is important. Often, health-care workers have to deal with withdrawal states and overdose. In addition, substance use can complicate HIV treatment among DUs by interfering with adherence and hence efforts should be made to link users requiring ART with drug treatment services (substitution treatment) to stabilize them. Irrespective of their continued use of illicit drugs, healthcare workers should strive to reduce drug-related harm in them by adopting harm-reduction strategies in prevention and care settings. These include OST, prevention and management of drug overdose, and prevention of HIV transmission through needle–syringe and condom programmes.

2.5.2.1 Harm-reduction approaches to managing injection drug-related harm

Rather than stigmatizing substance users, a harm-reduction approach recognizes that people who use drugs do so as a result of complex social, environmental, economic, cultural and personal factors often beyond their control.

Harm reduction involves a variety of strategies to reduce physical and social harm where complete abstinence is an unrealistic, difficult-to-achieve goal.

These strategies include a broad range of programmes such as:
- Accurate and credible information about safe injecting practices
- Access to new sterile injecting equipment through needle and syringe programmes
- Provision of primary health care
- Evidence-based drug dependence treatments, including OST.

Risk-reduction approaches for IDUs

The risk of bloodborne virus (BBV) transmission can be reduced by:
- Offering effective drug treatment such as OST
- Linking the patient with other social services
- Educating the patient on safer drug use:
  - Avoid injecting, use a different route of administration where possible.
  - Never reuse or share needles, water or drug preparation equipment.
  - Always use a sterile needle and syringe.
  - If this is not possible then clean injecting equipment thoroughly with bleach and water.
  - Use sterile water to prepare drugs for injecting.

- If this is not possible, use boiled water.
- Use a new or disinfected cooker and fresh cotton.
- Clean the injection site with a fresh alcohol swab.
- Safely dispose of needles after injecting.

Trust and credibility are important components of a strong patient–health-care worker relationship. A strong relationship can improve treatment outcomes. Harm-reduction programmes have often already established trust and credibility with DUs and hence are useful to work with in order to improve treatment and care of HIV-positive DUs.

2.5.2.2 Harm-reduction strategies for non-injecting opioid users

Non-injecting opioid users are at risk for transitioning to injecting and hence all opioid users should be targeted for harm reduction. Environmental and structural factors such as repressive drug law enforcement policies, increasing cost of drugs such as heroin and easy availability of injectable pharmaceuticals contribute to the transition to injecting drug use in South and South-East Asia.

Though there are few evidence-based approaches to prevent or delay transition from non-injecting to injecting, it is critical that information regarding the adverse consequences of injecting should be provided through outreach and on-site education to all drug-using populations. Opioid substitution is also appropriate in the context of non-injecting opioid dependence.

2.5.2.3 Harm-reduction strategies for amphetamine users

Educate and counsel ATS users

- Educate, advise and counsel ATS users on the possible adverse effects of ATS, even in low doses.
- Discourage concomitant alcohol and other drug use.
- Make users aware of the strategies to reduce health risks such as drinking appropriate amounts of water while using ATS.
- Avoid certain venues such as a dance party as this can exacerbate physiological risks, particularly through increased body heat and dehydration.

- All users must be encouraged to practise safe sexual behaviours.
- Discuss the risk-reduction plan with the substance user.
- Carry out brief interventions to alert users to the adverse consequences.

2.5.2.4 Diagnosis and assessment of substance use

Any diagnosis of dependent substance use should always be preceded by an assessment. This should include: a review of the substances used, presence of dependence, medical and psychiatric comorbidities, other important psychosocial factors, withdrawal symptoms, overdose history and HIV risk.

Substance use and dependence
- Quantity and frequency (including pattern) of use of all licit and illicit drugs
- Failed treatment and complications (e.g. overdose, detoxification)

Harmful use: clear evidence that the use of substances was responsible for psychological or physical harm to the user.

Dependent use: Three or more criteria (ICD-10) are required (exhibited during the past year) for a diagnosis of dependence:[43]
- strong desire to take the substance
- difficulty in controlling substance-taking behaviour (levels of use, onset, termination)
- withdrawal state (symptoms on stopping or reducing the intake)
- tolerance (increasing the quantity of the substance to get the same effect)
- neglect of other interests due to substance use
- persistent use despite evidence for substance use-related harm.

Medical and psychiatric comorbidities
Common medical problems in DUs include injection-related injuries and infections, viral hepatitis, TB, HIV and poor nutrition. These are discussed elsewhere in the document.

Psychiatric disorders include depression, anxiety and psychosis (*see* section 2.5.1 on Psychiatric disorders).

Psychosocial factors
These include difficulties with accommodation, issues with law enforcement, lack of employment and consistent income, and unstable personal relationships. DUs are often excluded from their own families.

It is important to give DUs a realistic expectation of the goals that can be achieved with treatment.

2.5.2.5 Withdrawal
Withdrawal symptoms are generally the opposite of the intoxication state.

Table 17. Symptoms and signs of opioid withdrawal

Symptoms	Observable signs
Nausea	Increased blood pressure
Muscle aches	Increased pulse rate
Abdominal cramps	Increased temperature
Irritability	Piloerection (goosebumps)
Loss of appetite	Increased pupil size
Weakness	Rhinorrhoea
Restlessness	Lacrimation
Headache	Tremor
Dizziness	Insomnia
Sneezing	Diarrhoea
Hot and cold flashes	Vomiting
Craving	Sweating
Yawning	

Alcohol withdrawal symptoms
The severity of alcohol withdrawal symptoms depends on the quantity and frequency of alcohol use. Symptoms begin within hours after the last drink and, in severe cases, progress to a peak 2–3 days later. Common symptoms of withdrawal are nausea, tremor, paroxysmal sweats, anxiety, agitation, tactile disturbances, visual disturbances, auditory disturbances (illusions and hallucinations) and headache. In severe cases, there may be disorientation, confusion and seizures.

Benzodiazepine withdrawal symptoms
Like alcohol and opioids, the severity of withdrawal symptoms depends on the

quantity, frequency and chronicity of use. Common symptoms are agitation, irritability, sweating, poor sleep, sensory changes such as heightened sensitivity to noise, light, smell and touch, muscle pains and twitching, depressed mood and anxiety or panic attacks. In severe cases, there may be hallucinations and seizures.

ATS withdrawal symptoms
Common symptoms are irritability, depressed mood, restlessness and agitation, fear, drowsiness and sleep disturbances.

Management of withdrawal

Management of withdrawal should be with the patient's consent and planned in advance. The withdrawal management plan should be jointly agreed to by the patient and clinician, with the clinician explaining the benefits, risks and discomforts that are expected during the withdrawal phase. Forced treatment is not recommended and is often not effective. At times, however, the PHCS team will be faced with having to treat an acute withdrawal state as an emergency.

It should be emphasized that treatment for withdrawal of opioid and other drug dependence is unlikely to result in cessation of drug use, particularly if the many concomitant psychosocial issues have not been resolved. If this is the case in a patient with opioid dependence, substitution therapy is recommended.

■ Treatment objectives

The treatment goals are
- Stabilization
- Reducing drug-related harm
- Improvement in health, social and occupational functioning
- Improvement in the quality of life
- Abstinence.

Acute withdrawal symptoms of alcohol and other drug use should be recognized and treated promptly, particularly in heavily dependent individuals.

Common health problems associated with drug use/injecting drug use

Alcohol withdrawal can be effectively managed with long half-life benzodiazepines such as diazepam. Severe withdrawal states characterized by delirium, fits and severe agitation need to be referred to drug treatment services or general medical services for management. Thiamine should be given intramuscularly in chronically dependent patients as it is more effectively absorbed in the early stage of withdrawal. For further information, refer to *Treatment and care for HIV-positive injecting drug users (module 5)* (ASEAN/USAID/WHO/FHI, 2007).[44]

There is little evidence on what constitutes effective management of *amphetamine withdrawal*. Treatment should be geared to reducing symptoms and diazepam or major tranquillizers can be used for this. For further information, refer to *Treatment and care for HIV-positive injecting drug users (module 5)* (ASEAN/USAID/WHO/FHI, 2007).[44]

Withdrawal from opioids is best managed with buprenorphine or methadone. Both can be used for treating withdrawal in an outpatient setting. Non-opioid withdrawal can be managed alternatively with clonidine/lofexidine (along with symptomatic treatment of pain and other symptoms) if methadone or buprenorphine are not available. For further information, refer to *Treatment and care for HIV-positive injecting drug users (module 4)* (ASEAN/USAID/WHO/FHI, 2007).[45]

Benzodiazepine withdrawal is best managed by getting the person to convert to diazepam using a benzodiazepine conversion chart and then gradually reducing the dose over a number of weeks. Rapid withdrawal from benzodiazepines can result in severe agitation, aggression and seizures. For further information, refer to *Treatment and care for HIV-positive injecting drug users (module 5)* (ASEAN/USAID/WHO/FHI, 2007).[44]

Table 18. Management of withdrawal

Substance	Medications for withdrawal	Psychosocial interventions	Pharmacotherapy for chronic dependence	Key issues
Alcohol	Tapered diazepam regimen Thiamine 100 mg IM or orally for at least 3 days	Brief interventions Cognitive–behavioural therapy Relapse prevention strategies Alcoholics Anonymous	Naltrexone Acamprosate	Continued engagement and retention is crucial
Amphetamines	Tapered diazepam regimen	Brief interventions Cognitive–behavioural therapy	Controversial and lacking effectiveness	Little evidence for effective treatment strategies
Opioids	Buprenorphine Methadone Clonidine/lofexidine-based regimen	Brief interventions	Buprenorphine Methadone	Opioid substitution therapy is the most effective
Benzodiazepines	Tapered diazepam regimen	Brief interventions Cognitive–behavioural therapy Relapse prevention strategies	Diazepam maintenance (though currently controversial)	Maintenance is effective though engagement in the treatment process is crucial

2.5.2.6 Management of substance dependence

Opioid substitution therapy

Opioid dependence is best managed with OST. For detailed management of opioid dependence with OST please refer to *Operational guidelines for the management of opioid dependence in the South-East Asia Region* (WHO, 2008).[46] The choice of methadone or buprenorphine generally depends on clinician and patient preference, though buprenorphine may be superior in higher-functioning individuals while methadone may be suited to those with concomitant psychiatric conditions such as psychosis, or those who prefer a greater sedative effect.

Table 19. Drugs used for opioid substitution therapy

Medication	Initial dose	Minimal time between dose increases	Maintenance dose	Duration of treatment
Methadone	20–30 mg daily Oral liquid	3 days (max. 10 mg each time)	>60 mg daily	Minimum of one year
Buprenorphine	2–4 mg daily Sublingual tablet	1 day	8–16 mg daily	Minimum of one year Transfer to other abstinence-oriented treatment following OST with buprenorphine is possible

Fluctuating levels of heroin while pregnant can harm the unborn child, reduce fetal growth and cause premature labour and stillbirth. Withdrawal symptoms from opioid dependence can occur in the newly born child. These are generally mild and do not require medical intervention in at least 75% of neonates. Pregnant opioid-dependent DUs should be considered a priority for drug substitution with methadone, rather than advocating withdrawal.

Sudden withdrawal from opioid dependence may precipitate miscarriage or premature labour.[47]

Pharmacotherapy for alcohol dependence
Maintenance of alcohol abstinence or reduced use can be enhanced by the use of naltrexone or acamprosate, both of which reduce the craving associated with withdrawal from alcohol. Although naltrexone is more effective in reducing relapse to alcohol use it cannot be used during OST nor should it be used in heroin users as it blocks the effects of opiates. In these cases, acamprosate should be used. Pharmacotherapy to reduce the chances of relapse should be given in conjunction with psychosocial interventions and support.

Management of acute ATS toxicity
Acute ATS toxicity with any of the following symptoms should be immediately referred for treatment:
- Chest pain
- Rapidly increasing body temperature
- Psychotic features
- Behaviour that is dangerous to self or others
- Seizures
- Uncontrolled hypertension (headache, dizziness, nausea)
- Exhaustion, insomnia.

Urgent sedation may be indicated for extreme behavioural disturbance associated with toxicity or if the patient is psychotic. In an emergency, treat with injection haloperidol.

Psychosocial interventions
A variety of psychosocial interventions are available that can be used for the treatment of substance use disorders. Some are more effective than others. These include:
- Brief interventions[48]
  - Providing patients with information on substance use and treatment options in a non-threatening, empathetic way

- Providing information and *feedback* about the risks of substance use; emphasizing *responsibility* in choosing less harmful substance use; providing a *menu* of treatment options; using *empathy* to engage the patient; engendering *self-efficacy*, the belief that things can be changed to enhance motivation
- Cognitive–behavioural therapy[45]
  - Is based on the link between beliefs and actions. If beliefs and thought patterns on drug use are changed, then a patient's pattern of drug use will change too. Training in good communication techniques to avoid situations that place pressure on the patient's often poor coping skills is a key component of this.
  - Needs to be performed by a trained clinician.
  - Is effective, but treatment requires a number of sessions over a period of time.
- Relapse-prevention strategies
  - Is based on the premise that high-risk environments are conducive to substance use. It seeks to delay and reduce the severity of relapse to substance use.
  - The patient works with the clinician to identify those factors that are most responsible for substance use and relapse, and structures their life to avoid putting themselves in these high-risk situations, e.g. avoiding a peer group that uses drugs when trying to reduce drug use.
  - May require long-term engagement
- Self-help groups
  - Are not expensive and can help in providing an empathetic environment for DUs who often suffer from substantial social exclusion
  - Are generally not effective in reducing substance use.

Psychosocial interventions depend on continued engagement with the client. Generally, the longer the patient is in treatment, the more effective the intervention. The type of psychosocial intervention is probably less important. Psychosocial treatments are generally not as effective as pharmacological treatments. Much depends on the quality of the patient–clinician relationship and the skills of the clinician working with the patient. Confidentiality and trust are crucial.

2.5.2.7 Overdose
Heroin overdose*

Heroin use is associated with a significant increase in mortality. Approximately half of the mortality is due to overdose. The risk of overdose may be as high as 2% per year. Heroin overdose is characterized by respiratory depression, which may lead to death. Death usually occurs 1–3 hours after injection rather than suddenly.

The most common scenarios for a significant heroin overdose are the use of a higher dose, the accidental injection of highly concentrated solution, or the use of heroin after a prolonged period of abstinence. Intentional (i.e. suicidal) overdoses are rare.

- ■ **Symptoms of heroin overdose**
- Muscle spasticity
- Slow, laboured and shallow breathing
- Respiratory arrest (sometimes fatal within 2–4 hours)
- Pinpoint pupils
- Dry mouth
- Cold and clammy skin
- Tongue discolouration
- Bluish-coloured fingernails and lips
- Spasms of the stomach and/or intestinal tract
- Constipation
- Weak pulse
- Low blood pressure
- Drowsiness
- Disorientation
- Coma
- Delirium

---

*Risk factors, symptoms and management of overdose for methadone, morphine and other opioids are generally similar to those of heroin.

Common health problems associated with drug use/injecting drug use

- **Risk factors for heroin overdose**
- Using heroin for 5–10 years
- Recent release from detoxification or correctional facility
- Street-based injecting
- Using heroin when alone
- Mixing heroin with alcohol or benzodiazepines
- Concurrent serious medical conditions, particularly pulmonary and hepatic dysfunction
- Previous history of overdose
- Depression
- Poverty and homelessness
- Poor social support
- Changing one's source of heroin

- **Prevention and management of heroin overdose**

Primary health-care providers should counsel substance-using patients about the risk of overdose and how it may be prevented.

Patients should be taught the following:
- The risks of mixing sedative drugs with heroin
- The risk of reinitiating heroin use after a period of abstinence
- The risk of using opioids/drugs when alone
- To recognize the signs of a possible heroin overdose in another user and to immediately call for medical help (many people who overdose are not alone)
- OST is an effective long-term preventive strategy for overdose.

OVERDOSE DON'TS
- Don't leave the person alone by themselves – they could stop breathing.
- Don't throw the person in a bath – they could drown.
- Don't make the person try to vomit – they could aspirate their vomit.
- Don't give the person something to drink – this may cause them to vomit or aspirate the drink.
- Don't inject anything into the person (unless it is naloxone) – they need help, not more drugs or salt or water.

Naloxone can be stored at the PHCS in areas where heroin use is common. Naloxone can be given IM or IV during overdose. Training in cardiopulmonary resuscitation (CPR) is essential for primary care workers and outreach workers (Figure 11).[49]

Figure 11. Steps for cardiopulmonary resuscitation in a patient with overdose

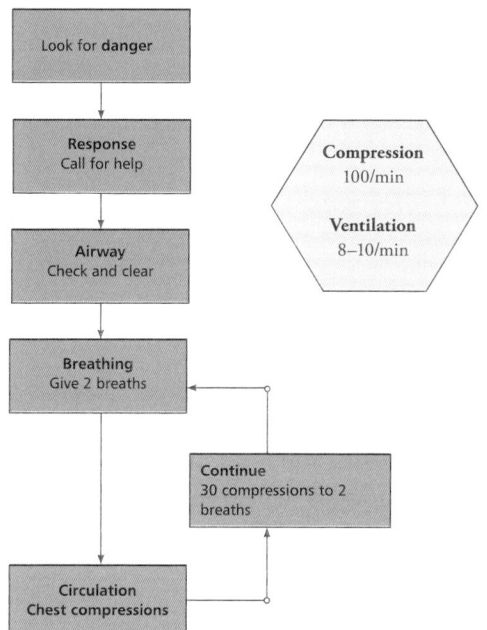

2.6 Other common medical problems

2.6.1 Pain

Drug users have higher rates of injury/trauma which can cause pain. At the same time, chronic opioid users can develop a tolerance to opioid effects. Therefore, it is incorrect to assume that individuals who are opioid-dependent should receive less pain medication because they are dependent. Analgesia should be sufficient to provide relief from pain. This may require significantly higher doses of analgesics than might normally be required.

Appropriate actions to treat DUs in acute pain related to a recent diagnosable injury involve the following:

- Determine the source of the pain.
- Provide appropriate pain medication to relieve the symptoms; this may include opioids.
- Analgesia should be prescribed on a regular basis. Additional flexibility for "breakthrough" pain may be required.
- If the pain is persistent or the cause is unclear, check for underlying psychiatric problems or an undetected source of pain.
- If opioids are used, opioid-dependent users require more and frequent doses of narcotic analgesics compared with non-dependent users due to their tolerance.
- In methadone-maintained patients receiving opioid analgesics, these should be given in addition to the daily maintenance dose of methadone (perhaps even at a higher dose).
- Taper the doses of narcotic analgesics slowly to avoid drug withdrawal.

If the pain is chronic, the treatment strategies are:
- finding the source of the pain
- using the entire spectrum of pain-relieving strategies, including using combinations of analgesics with different mechanisms of action.

2.6.1.1 Pharmacotherapy for pain management

Treating chronic pain in known DUs
- Paracetamol (rule out hepatic impairment before administration)
- Other non-opioid analgesics such as NSAIDs or aspirin
- Opioids starting with combinations of codeine/NSAID or paracetamol or tramadol (use with caution in clients on OST)

Treating neuropathic pain
- Anticonvulsants
- Antidepressants
- Benzodiazepines

For further information, refer to *Treatment and care for HIV-infected injecting drug users: module 10* (ASEAN/USAID/WHO/FHI, 2007).[50]

Table 19. Medication for pain control in drug users

Intensity/nature of pain	Drug used	Dosage and recommendation
Mild pain	NSAIDs *Ibuprofen*	400–800 mg tid Contraindicated in patients with gastrointestinal bleeding and/or bleeding disorders. Use with caution in patients with liver disease.
	Aspirin (acetylsalicylic acid)	325–500 mg every 4 hours up to a total of 2 g Contraindicated in patients with gastrointestinal bleeding and/or bleeding disorders. Use with caution in patients with liver disease.
	Paracetamol	650 mg 4 hourly Use with careful monitoring in patients with liver disease; toxicity is dose-related.
Moderate pain	Oral codeine	25–50 mg every 4 hours Prevent constipation through use of a stool softener and bowel stimulant, use laxatives if needed.
	Tramadol	50–100 mg every 6 hours
	± non-opioids (aspirin/ paracetamol/ ibuprofen	
Severe pain	Oral morphine	10–20 mg every 3–4 hours in tablet or liquid form Prevent constipation through use of a stool softener and bowel stimulant, use laxatives if needed
	Oral oxycodone	5–10 mg every 4 hours
	± non-opioids (aspirin/ paracetamol/ ibuprofen	

Intensity/nature of pain	Drug used	Dosage and recommendation
Neuropathic pain	Carbamazepine* Amitriptyline	200–400 mg every 6 hours 25 mg at night

*In patients on OST, plasma levels of methadone may be reduced by carbamazepine and hence dose adjustment of methadone may be required as clinically indicated. Carbamazepine can also interact with efavirenz, lopinavir and nevirapine, and should be used with caution in patients on ARVs.

Doses suggested are the starting doses for moderating severe pain in opioid-naive adults ≥50 kg.

- Good pain management uses combinations of analgesics to treat pain effectively. Opioids should be used when pain is refractory to paracetamol or NSAIDs.
- Opioid-dependent persons due to their tolerance to opioids require increased as well as frequent doses.
- Pain management for IDUs is the same as for non-IDUs, only the dose of the analgesic needed is usually higher.
- In the case of OST, the substitution dose should be maintained and opioid analgesics added. A splitting of the OST dose should be considered as the analgesic effect of methadone vanishes after 6–8 hours.

Source: Adapted from *Palliative care for people living with HIV/AIDS: clinical protocols for the WHO European Region* (WHO, 2006)[51] and *HIV/AIDS treatment and care: clinical protocols for the WHO European Region* (WHO 2007).[22]

2.6.1.2 Non-pharmacological interventions
- Thermal: heat and cold are both effective and underutilized.
- Manual therapies: massage, and chiropractic and osteopathic manipulation
- Active movement: stretching and active exercises
- Orthotics: splints and other supportive devices
- Acupuncture (where available)

2.6.2 Constipation

Constipation is relatively common among opioid users.
- Primary prevention strategies
  - Increased dietary fibre
  - Increased fluid intake
  - Adequate exercise
  - Adequate time and privacy for going to the toilet

Patients on opioids may require the help of pharmacological agents as primary prevention strategies alone may not suffice. However, they should always be counselled that long-term use of laxatives can be hazardous.

Types of pharmacological agents available for the treatment of constipation:
- Osmotic laxatives (e.g. lactulose, sorbitol, milk of magnesia)
- Emollient or lubricant cathartics (e.g. glycerine suppositories)
- Stool softeners (e.g. docusate)
- Bulk laxatives (e.g. psyllium seed husk)

If the patient has faecal impaction, an enema may be the only way to break up the hardened faecal matter. Once the impaction has been removed, enemas should be used sparingly since they tend to wash out the normal mucus in the colon, which provides lubrication for stools.

2.6.3 Poor dental condition

Many drug-dependent individuals neglect their dental health before, and at times even after, entering intervention programmes. It is necessary to assess the dental health and refer them for appropriate treatment.

■ Risk factors

Dental problems are often seen in opioid and ATS users. Poor dental health is related to teeth grinding (particularly associated with ATS use), reduced saliva secretion and not brushing. Poor dental health can increase the risk of bacteraemia and infective endocarditis. Xerostomia, which can be a side-effect of methadone, can contribute to a high rate of caries.

Oral lesions in HIV-positive DUs include:
- candidiasis
- oral hairy leukoplakia
- HIV-associated gingivitis
- HIV-associated periodontitis
- necrotizing ulcerative gingivitis and gingivostomatitis
- recurrent herpes simplex
- bacterial glossitis
- major aphthous ulcers
- molluscum contagiosum
- patchy depapillated tongue
- hairy tongue
- angular cheilitis.

■ Treatment

PHCS workers have to advise patients on proper dental care and the advantages of dental check-up and treatment. Referral linkages have to be established with the dental health services to provide adequate care for DUs with and without HIV infection. DUs continuing to use opiates or on OST should be encouraged to chew sugar-free gum and brush teeth regularly to improve dental health.

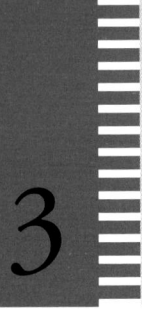

3 Universal precautions in the primary health-care setting

3.1 Universal precautions

These are simple infection control measures that reduce the risk of transmission of bloodborne pathogens through exposure to blood or body fluids among patients and health-care workers.

- It is important to follow universal precautions in health-care settings.
- Health care-associated infections are preventable.
- Improving the safety of injections is an important component of universal precautions.
- Blood and body fluids are primary sources of HIV infection in health-care settings.
- Infection can be transmitted by blood or body fluids in direct contact with an open wound.
- A prick with an infected needle or sharp stick can also transmit infection.

Under the "universal precautions" principle, blood and body fluids from all persons should be considered as infected with HIV regardless of the known or supposed status of the person. For further information, refer to *Management of HIV infection and antiretroviral therapy in adults and adolescents: a clinical manual* (WHO, 2007).[35]

3.2 Post-exposure prophylaxis (PEP)

3.2.1 Management of PEP

Refer to the national guidelines on PEP.

PRACTICAL POINTS

Do	Do not
Remove gloves, if appropriate	Do not panic
Wash the exposed site thoroughly with running water	Do not put pricked finger in mouth
Irrigate with water or saline if exposure sites are eyes or mouth	Do not squeeze wound to bleed it
Wash skin with soap and water	Do not use bleach, chlorine, alcohol, betadine, iodine or other antiseptics/detergents on the wound

Do – Consult the designated physician immediately as per institutional guidelines for the management of occupational exposure.

Annexes

Annex 1

Principles for establishing services for drug users
How do primary health-care services retain patients in care?
- Respect, cultural competence: Respecting patients, being culturally sensitive and providing them with effective care builds trust and keeps them coming back.
- Welcoming attitude of staff: Patients should always be made to feel that they have come to the right place. Many clinics employ persons from the target community and they help patients ask questions or make their needs known to clinical staff.
- Welcoming environment: Physically comfortable waiting and examination areas, with linguistically and culturally appropriate decoration and reading material, are important for patient retention.
- Orientation to clinic systems and rules: New patients need a brief description of clinic staff and services, routine and emergency procedures, specific treatment procedures and after-hours follow up. Patients must also be oriented as to what is expected of them (e.g. coming on time, informing the clinic in the event of cancellation or rescheduling of appointments) and the consequences of not fulfilling their responsibilities (e.g. rules regarding late arrival, violent/unruly behaviour on the premises).

How to establish and maintain a follow-up mechanism
Every clinic should
- be linked to agencies providing HIV testing and services for persons with HIV.
- make clinic access easy for the clients of outside services.

Clinics shall establish referral linkages with community services such as:
- HIV testing and counselling services
- AIDS service organizations (ASOs)
- STI treatment facilities
- Family planning agencies
- Drug treatment facilities
- Local health departments
- Regional HIV/AIDS services
- Local and general hospitals
- Emergency medical services
- TB clinics.

Mobilizing community support
- Clinics should target a narrow but underserved population and concentrate on meeting the needs of that population.
- Advocacy targeting the general community is required to establish and operate services for DUs.
- In order to sustain the services, PHCS have to advocate to, and work closely with, community leaders, government agencies (health and public security) and donor agencies.

Policies and procedures
There should be specific policies and procedures regarding the operation of the PHCS. All staff must be trained in following these policies.
These should include:
- Specific measures taken to protect patient confidentiality;
- Procedure to be followed for late arrival or non-attendance of clients at clinic appointments
  - A patient's right to accept or refuse treatment should be respected and, as such, clients who do not attend an appointment should not be followed up without their express consent.
  - If the PHCS is to be involved in the daily dosing of patients on DOT for TB or ART, they should establish policies for clients who do not attend for dosing. Consent by the patient to be contacted by clinic staff

     following non-attendance should be obtained prior to commencement of treatment.
- Addressing TB prevention and risk assessment for all staff of the PHCS;
- Occupational health and safety issues, especially related to the disposal of used injecting equipment;
- Procedure in the event of a needle-stick injury, especially PEP for HIV/AIDS;
- Recommending immunization of staff against HBV and tetanus;
- A clear statement that staff must not be involved in the procurement or distribution of illicit substances to, or from, patients of the PHCS;
- Performance management and supervision of staff;
- Clear guidelines on grievance procedures for both staff and patients to address management of conflict, should it arise;
- Who can access the PHCS. Provision of services to PHCS staff and their families should be considered. Access should also be extended to partners and family members of DUs/IDUs, as well as the local community, but not at the expense of access by DUs/IDUs;
- Ongoing training to maintain and upgrade clinical and technical skills. It is important that all staff is offered, and have access to, regular in-service education and training.

Annex 2

Operational issues: staff, facilities and equipment
PHCS staff

Service providers from a range of backgrounds (medicine, nursing, social work and others) may be involved in providing primary health care. The roles and mix of staff will vary according to geographical areas, qualifications, programme settings and available resources. Ideally, a suggested mix of staff with the relevant qualifications* could include:

1. **Service coordinator** or **programme manager** with qualifications in public health, good management skills and knowledge of the behavioural/social sciences. They would have overall responsibility for all aspects of the drop-in centre (DIC), including the PHCS;
2. **Medical officer** (part-time) with a recognized license. Some PHCS programmes may have limited resources. Although the presence of an on-site MO is optimal, operationally it may not always be possible. Basic health care can be provided at the clinic by nurses or health workers. Clients with more pressing health needs may be referred to a local hospital or general practitioner's clinic;
3. **Registered nurse** with a university degree or diploma in nursing with experience in clinic work or community health services;
4. **Counsellor** – trained and experienced in counselling;
5. **Health worker** – trained and experienced in basic health care, infection control and simple dressing techniques;
6. **Peer educator/outreach worker** – functions as a community health worker and patient advocate. Community health training and experience of

---

*These are not compulsory requirements, but rather requirements in an ideal setting.

working with IDUs is a minimum qualification; outreach staff could also be utilized to treat simple wounds, e.g. abscesses. Workers could then refer, and possibly accompany, clients with more advanced health needs to the PHCS for assessment or directly to a general practitioner's clinic or hospital;
7. **Administrative officer** responsible for maintaining records, managing information systems for proper monitoring and evaluation (part-time). Experience in administrative and managerial aspects, and proficiency in the use of computers are required; and
8. **Attendant** or security guard for the clinic.

The services could satisfactorily function with a registered nurse, peer educators/outreach workers and attendant/security guard.

Desirable characteristics of the staff
- Ability to make the DU feel welcome in the facility
- Ability to work as a clinical team and actively participate/contribute to team meetings
- Capacity to establish rapport with the clients
- Allowing the patients time and freedom to reflect on their drug use and related health concerns
- Ability to be open and non-judgemental to facilitate meaningful interaction with clients
- Respect for and empathy with clients
- Willingness to exchange information and ideas/thoughts
- Willingness to learn and enhance capacity to better manage clients.

Training and technical assistance

Patients look to non-technical staff to corroborate information given by physicians and paramedical staff. Further, patients expect the same accepting attitude from all staff members. Thus, all staff members need training in both technical and cultural matters. Training sessions, particularly to assist clinicians in making appropriate treatment decisions, are required. Written educational/training materials for staff, such as national and regional treatment guidelines, should be made available and frequently updated. Many regional and national meetings provide training in both clinical care and prevention, and primary care staff should be encouraged to attend these. Assistance with enhancing and implementing systems of care, including instituting a quality management programme, is also desirable. Close collaboration and coordination are needed between the primary care and the specialized HIV/AIDS care and treatment centre at the district/province level. Knowledgeable and sensitive health workers and others (peers) are needed to support vulnerable PLHIV and maintain harm-reduction activities. These workers and peers require ongoing training. All staff members require comprehensive training in various aspects relating to injecting drug use. These include:

- Safe injecting practices
- Vein care
- Safe sex practices
- Medical conditions associated with injecting drug use
- Medical conditions associated with HIV and TB infections
- Management and prevention of overdose
- Management of drug dependence-related issues;
- Infection control and universal precautions.

Staff members also require training and education on the importance of not imposing their own attitudes and beliefs regarding injecting drug use.

Supportive supervision and debriefing

Supportive supervision provides workers with the opportunity to actively review their work practices and seek advice, structure and direction from a more experienced worker in a supportive environment. The aim is to support and develop workers in this role.

Debriefing is a supportive process which offers staff an informal opportunity to express their feelings, thoughts and reactions about an unpleasant, negative or difficult work experience to a colleague or supervisor. It should be immediate, informal and low key, and is an important component of preventing staff burn-out. Debriefing promotes teamwork and trust among team members. It also promotes skill-sharing and an opportunity to review work practices.

Annexes

Facilities and equipment

In addition to the usual clinic layout, other facilities are useful. An examination room suitable for private examination (e.g. gynaecological examination) is important.

Easy access to facilities for drawing blood, urine and stool specimens should be available. On-site access to rapid tests may be helpful (e.g. urine pregnancy tests, and rapid tests for syphilis and HIV).

Refrigeration for the maintenance and storage of vaccines and medicines is necessary. An autoclave or pressure cooker is required to sterilize instruments and other items.

Other equipment required for PHCS
- Stethoscope
- BP apparatus – sphygmomanometer
- Thermometer
- Torch
- Tongue depressor
- Weighing scales
- Kidney trays
- Alcohol swabs
- Dressing material (sterile gauze – wet and dry)
- Disposable gloves and masks
- Sterile gowns and boots
- Hydrogen peroxide solution
- Chlorhexidine antiseptic solution
- Solvent ether spirit, povidone iodine solution, freshly prepared 1% sodium hypochlorite solution, drums with sterilized instruments (e.g. Cheatle forceps), drums with sterile gauze and bandages, sterile packets of catgut and non-absorbable monofilament nylon/polypropylene sutures, autoclaved linen, sticking plaster, 2% lignocaine without adrenaline, suture-cutting scissors, disposable syringes (5, 10, 20 cc), disposable needles (curved, cutting and round-bodied) in small and medium sizes kept in antiseptic solution

- Examination table with mattress to carry out dressings and dressing trolley
- Wash basin with liquid soap dispenser and towel rail
- Stationery items
- Sachets for dispensing medicines
- Emergency medicine tray
- Essential drugs including naloxone for the management of overdose
- Ambu® bag resuscitator
- IV stands
- Test-tubes with stands
- Reagents for various tests
- Anticoagulants, preservatives
- Bedside microscope
- Storage bins for hazardous waste
- Emergency lights
- Back-up generator or solar/battery supply
- Educational materials

Annex 3

Antibiotics used to treat infections in drug users

Injection-related infections	Antibiotics
Cellulitis and abscesses	Cloxacillin: 250–500 mg x 4 times/day for 5 days Cefixime: 200 mg x 2 times/day for 5 days orally Ceftriaxone: 1 g given every 24 hours until erythema regresses followed by oral antibiotics IM*/IV
Thrombophlebitis	Cloxacillin: 250–500 mg x 4 times/day for 5 days Cefixime: 200 mg x 2 times/day for 5 days orally
Septicaemia	Cloxacillin plus gentamicin: cloxacillin 1–2 g /day; gentamicin 150–300 mg/day – IM*/IV Ceftriaxone: 1–2 g once daily – IM*/IV Duration dependent on severity
Septic arthritis Osteomyelitis	Cloxacillin 1–2 g/day – IM*/IV Ampicillin 1–2 g every 6 hours – IM*/IV and Gentamicin 150–300 mg/day – IM*/IV
Infective endocarditis	Cloxacillin plus gentamicin: cloxacillin 1–2 g/day; gentamicin 150–300 mg/day – IM*/IV Ampicillin 1 g x 3 plus gentamicin 1.5 ml of 160 mg ampoule x 2 Intravenous therapy for at least 4 weeks
Severe pneumonia	Cloxacillin plus gentamicin: cloxacillin 1–2 g/day; gentamicin 150–300 mg/day – IM*/IV Ceftriaxone: 1–2 g once daily – IM*/IV Clindamycin: 2400 mg/day in four divided doses at 6-hour intervals orally

Injection-related infections	Antibiotics
Aspiration pneumonia	Same as above and add metronidazole
Bronchitis	Amoxicillin (500 mg tablet: 2 tabs x twice daily for 7 days or inj. amoxicillin 1 g vial x 3 IM*/IV and change to oral treatment as soon as possible Ampicillin plus gentamicin (ampicillin 1 g vial x 3 IV plus gentamicin 1.5 ml of 160 mg ampoule x 2). Change to oral treatment as soon as possible
Upper respiratory tract infections	Amoxicillin (500 mg tablet: 1 tab x twice daily for 7 days) Erythromycin (2 g/day in 2–3 divided doses for 7 days) Azithromycin (500 mg once daily for 3 days)

*IM if there is difficulty in accessing a vein in IDUs.

Annex 4

Sample educational materials for injecting drug users
Preventing soft tissue infections
Infection is caused by
- Use of non-sterile needles
- Improper cleaning of the injection site
- Contamination from the solution in which the drug may be dissolved or the drug itself.

Reducing the occurrence of abscesses and cellulitis
- Dirty needles contribute to abscesses and should be avoided.
- IDUs who report cleaning their skin before injecting have a lower rate of abscesses.
- Abscesses are more likely in HIV-positive IDUs.
- Alcohol prep pads alone may not be sufficient to clean the injection site. Alcohol lacks the sustained residual antimicrobial activity of chlorhexidine and iodophors.
- Avoid the following risk factors:
  - skin-popping
  - mixing different preparations (for example, cocktails of diazepam, pheniramine maleate with buprenorphine injection)
  - frequent injecting and "booting" (repeatedly flushing and pulling back during injecting)
- Education about safe and sterile injection techniques could help IDUs preserve access to their veins and reduce the risk of infection associated with skin-popping.

- Targeted health services and early referral for treatment of abscesses and cellulitis reduces morbidity and the need for lengthy hospital admissions.
- Methadone treatment reduces hospital admissions related to abscesses and cellulitis.

Information on hepatitis
- Hepatitis B and C are serious viral infections that affect the liver.
- Both hepatitis B and C are transmitted by sharing injection equipment and paraphernalia.
- Hepatitis B is also transmitted by the sexual route.
- IDUs should be tested for hepatitis B and C.
- Vaccination is available for hepatitis B and is highly recommended for IDUs.
- Coinfection with HIV and hepatitis B or hepatitis C (or both) is quite common.
- Hepatitis B can make one ill in both the short- and the long term.
- Treatment is available for hepatitis B, some of which also works against HIV.
- Hepatitis C can cause serious long-term health problems.
- Hepatitis C is a major cause of illness and death in people with HIV.
- Those infected with hepatitis C and/or B must avoid alcohol.
- Treatment is available for hepatitis B and C.
- Treatment decisions should be made on an individual basis.

Information on hepatitis C
DO
- Find a doctor who understands HCV.
- Get vaccinated against hepatitis B and A if required.
- Get regular health check-ups.
- Consider stopping or reducing alcohol intake.
- Alcohol use *significantly* increases the risk of developing cirrhosis and liver cancer.
- Having hepatitis C antibodies *will not* protect one from becoming infected again.

- Stick to a balanced diet of fresh vegetables, fruits, beans, whole grains and lean meats.
- Get a healthy balance of protein in the diet.
- Drink lots of fluids to flush toxins from your body.
- Get regular exercise.
- Develop a stress reduction plan.

AVOID
- Drinking alcohol; even one drink a day can accelerate the progression of liver disease.
- Taking large amounts of acetaminophen is toxic to the liver.
- Together, acetaminophen and alcohol can cause severe liver damage.
- Breathing in pollutants, chemicals, cleaning products, fumes from paint, paint thinners, chemical solvents, spray adhesives, insect sprays and cleaners can be harmful to the liver.
- Foods with high salt, sugar or fat content can cause damage.
- Do not take too much of fried foods.
- High doses of vitamins A, D, E or K must not be taken.
- Iron supplements should not be taken unless advised by the doctor.

References

1. http://www.who.int/substance_abuse/terminology/who_lexicon/en/index.html (accessed on 15 September 2008).

2. Reid G, Costigan G. *Revisiting the "hidden epidemic": a situation assessment of drug use in Asia in the context of HIV/AIDS*. Melbourne, Australia, Centre for Harm Reduction, Burnet Institute, 2002.

3. Garten R et al. Rapid transmission of hepatitis C virus among young injecting heroin users in Southern China. *International Journal of Epidemiology*, 2004, 33:182–188.

4. Hammett M et al. Correlates of HIV status among injecting drug users in a border region of southern China and northern Viet Nam. *Journal of Acquired Immune Deficiency Syndromes*, 2005, 38:228–235.

5. Mith Samlanh – Friends. *Drug use and HIV vulnerability*. Phnom Penh, International HIV/AIDS Alliance, 2002.

6. Rahman Z et al. Drug sharing and injecting networks in Bangladesh: implications for HIV transmission. XV International AIDS Conference, 11–16 July 2004 (abstract no. C12531).

7. Lewis DR. *The long trip down the mountain: social and economic impacts of illicit drugs in Thailand*. Bangkok, UNODC, 2003.

8. Liu T, Hao W. *WHO multi-site project in amphetamine-type stimulants: evaluation report from China*. Geneva, World Health Organization, 2002.

References

[9] Kiatying-Angsulee N et al. Midazolam tablet injection in Bangkok: pattern of use and HIV risk behaviour. Poster for XV International AIDS Conference, 11–16 July 2004 Available at: http://gateway.nlm.nih.gov/meetingAbstracts/102283974.html (accessed on 28 August 2008).

[10] Tuan NA et al. Intravenous drug use among street-based sex workers: a high-risk behaviour for HIV transmission. *Sexually Transmitted Diseases*, 2004, 31:15–19.

[11] Monitoring the AIDS Pandemic (MAP) Network. *MAP report 2005: drug injection and HIV/AIDS in Asia*. Bangkok, MAP Network, 2005:9.

[12] Preamble to the Constitution of the World Health Organization as adopted by the International Health Conference, New York, 19–22 June, 1946; signed on 22 July 1946 by the representatives of 61 States (Official Records of the World Health Organization, no. 2, p. 100) and entered into force on 7 April 1948.

[13] The WHO/UNODC *Evidence for Action series and policy briefs*. Available at: http://www.who.int/hiv/pub/idu/en/

[14] Ball A, Weiler G, Beg M, Doupe A. Editorial. WHO Evidence for Action for HIV prevention, treatment and care among injecting drug users. *The International Journal of Drug Policy*, 2005, 16(1):S1–S6.

[15] Gordon RJ, Lowy FD. Bacterial infections in drug users. *New England Journal of Medicine*, 2005, 353:1945–1954.

[16] CDC. Tetanus among injecting drug users – California, 1997. *MMWR Morbidity and Mortality Weekly Report*, 1998, 47:149–151.

[17] WHO. *Guidelines for the management of sexually transmitted infections*. Geneva, WHO, 2003. Available at: http://www.who.int/hiv/pub/sti/en/STIGuidelines2003.pdf (accessed on 20 September 2008).

[18] WHO. *Regional guidelines for the management of sexually transmitted infections.* New Delhi, WHO Regional Office for South-East Asia, 2007 (draft).

[19] WHO. *Sexually transmitted and other reproductive tract infections: a guide to essential practice.* Geneva, WHO, 2005.

[20] ASEAN/USAID/WHO/FHI. *Treatment and care for HIV-positive injecting drug users: management of coinfections in HIV-positive injecting drug users (module 9).* Jakarta, ASEAN/USAID/WHO/FHI, 2007.

[21] Aceijas C, Rhodes T. Global estimates of prevalence of HCV infection among injecting drug users. *International Journal on Drug Policy,* 2007, 18:352–358.

[22] WHO. *HIV/AIDS treatment and care: clinical protocols for the WHO European Region.* Copenhagen, WHO Regional Office for Europe, 2007.

[23] http://www.who.int/hiv/topics/tb/en/index.html (accessed on 10 September 2008).

[24] WHO. *Global tuberculosis control 2008. Surveillance, planning, financing.* Geneva, WHO, 2008.

[25] WHO. *Tuberculosis care with TB–HIV co-management. Integrated Management of Adolescent and Adult Illnesses* (IMAI). Geneva, WHO, 2007.

[26] WHO. *Guidance on testing and counselling for HIV in settings attended by people who inject drugs: improving access to treatment, care and prevention.* Manila, WHO Regional Office for the Western Pacific, 2009.

[27] Pallela FJ et al. Declining morbidity and mortality among patients with advanced human immunodeficiency virus infection. HIV Outpatient Study Investigators. *New England Journal of Medicine*, 1998, 338:853–860.

References

[28] Press N, Tyndall MW, Wood E. Virologic and immunologic response, clinical progression, and highly active antiretroviral therapy adherence. *Journal of Acquired Immune Deficiency Syndromes*, 2003, 31:5112–5117.

[29] Mocroft A et al. Changing patterns of mortality across Europe in patients infected with HIV-1. *Lancet*, 1998, 352:1725–30.

[30] Dore GJ et al. Impact of highly active antiretroviral therapy on individual AIDS-defining illness incidence and survival in Australia. *J AIDS*, 2002, 29:388–395.

[31] Currier JS et al. Incidence rates and risk factors for opportunistic infections in a phase III trial comparing indinavir + ZDV + 3TC to ZDV + 3TC. 5th Conference on Retroviruses and Opportunistic infections, 1–5 February 1998 [Abstract].

[32] WHO. *Guidelines on co-trimoxazole prophylaxis for HIV-related infections among children, adolescents and adults in resource-limited settings: recommendations for a public health approach.* Geneva, World Health Organization, 2006.

[33] Fornal F et al. Systematic review of the safety of trimethoprim–sulfamethoxazole for prophylaxis in HIV-infected pregnant women: implications for resource-limited settings. *AIDS Reviews*, 2006, 8:24.

[34] Walter J et al. Co-trimoxazole prophylaxis and adverse birth outcomes among HIV-infected women in Lusaka, Zambia. 13th Conference on Retroviruses and Opportunistic Infections, February 2006, Denver, Colorado. Abstract 126.

[35] WHO. *Management of HIV infection and antiretroviral therapy in adults and adolescents: a clinical manual.* New Delhi, WHO Regional Office for South-East Asia, 2007.

[36] Furrer H et al. Discontinuation of primary prophylaxis against *Pneumocystis carinii* pneumonia in HIV-1-infected adults treated with combination antiretroviral therapy. *New England Journal of Medicine*, 1999, 340:1301–1306.

[37] Kumarasamy N et al. Safe discontinuation of primary *Pneumocystis* prophylaxis in South Indian HIV-infected patients on HAART. *Journal of Acquired Immune Deficiency Syndromes*, 2005, 40:377–378.

[38] Robertson J et al. Immune reconstitution syndrome in HIV: validating a case definition and identifying clinical predictors in persons initiating antiretroviral therapy. *Clinical Infectious Diseases*, 2006, 42:1639–1646.

[39] Lipman M, Breen R. Immune reconstitution inflammatory syndrome in HIV. *Current Opinion in Infectious Diseases*, 2006,19:20–25.

[40] French MA et al. Immune restoration disease after the treatment of immunodeficient HIV-infected patients with highly active antiretroviral therapy. *HIV Medicine*, 2000, 1:107–115.

[41] Breen RAM et al. Paradoxical reactions during tuberculosis treatment in patients with and without HIV co-infection. *Thorax*, 2004, 59:704–707.

[42] ASEAN/USAID/WHO/FHI. *Treatment and care for HIV-positive drug users: managing ART in injecting drug users (module 6.5)*. Jakarta, ASEAN/USAID/WHO/FHI, 2007.

[43] WHO. *ICD-10 symptom checklist for mental disorders: psychoactive substance use syndromes module*. Geneva, WHO, 2004.

[44] ASEAN/USAID/WHO/FHI. *Treatment and care for HIV-positive injecting drug users: management of coinfections in HIV-positive injecting drug users (module 5)*. Jakarta, ASEAN/USAID/WHO/FHI, 2007.

References

[45] ASEAN/USAID/WHO/FHI. *Treatment and care for HIV-positive injecting drug users: management of coinfections in HIV-positive injecting drug users (module 4).* Jakarta, ASEAN/USAID/WHO/FHI, 2007.

[46] WHO. *Operational guidelines for the management of opioid dependence in the South-East Asia Region.* New Delhi, WHO Regional Office for South-East Asia, 2008.

[47] New South Wales Department of Health. *National clinical guidelines for the management of drug use during pregnancy, birth and the early development years of the newborn.* Sydney, NSW Department of Health, 2008.

[48] WHO. *Brief intervention for substance use: a manual for use in primary care.* Geneva, WHO, 2005. Available at: http://www.who.int/substance_abuse/activities/en/Draft_Brief_Intervention_for_Substance_Use.pdf (accessed on 28 August 2008).

[49] 2005 American Heart Association Guidelines for cardiopulmonary resuscitation and emergency cardiovascular care: overview of CPR. *Circulation*, 2005, 112:IV-12–IV-18.

[50] ASEAN/USAID/WHO/FHI. *Treatment and care for HIV-infected injecting drug users: managing pain in HIV-infected drug users (module 10).* Jakarta, ASEAN/USAID/WHO/FHI, 2007.

[51] WHO. *Palliative care for people living with HIV/AIDS: clinical protocols for the WHO European Region.* Copenhagen, WHO Regional Office for the European Region, 2006.